Marvelous Mary

Deaf with Cochlear Implants

by Mary & Emily Christensen
editing & design by Nathan Christensen

HWC
PRESS

Hi! My name is Mary, and I'm marvelous!

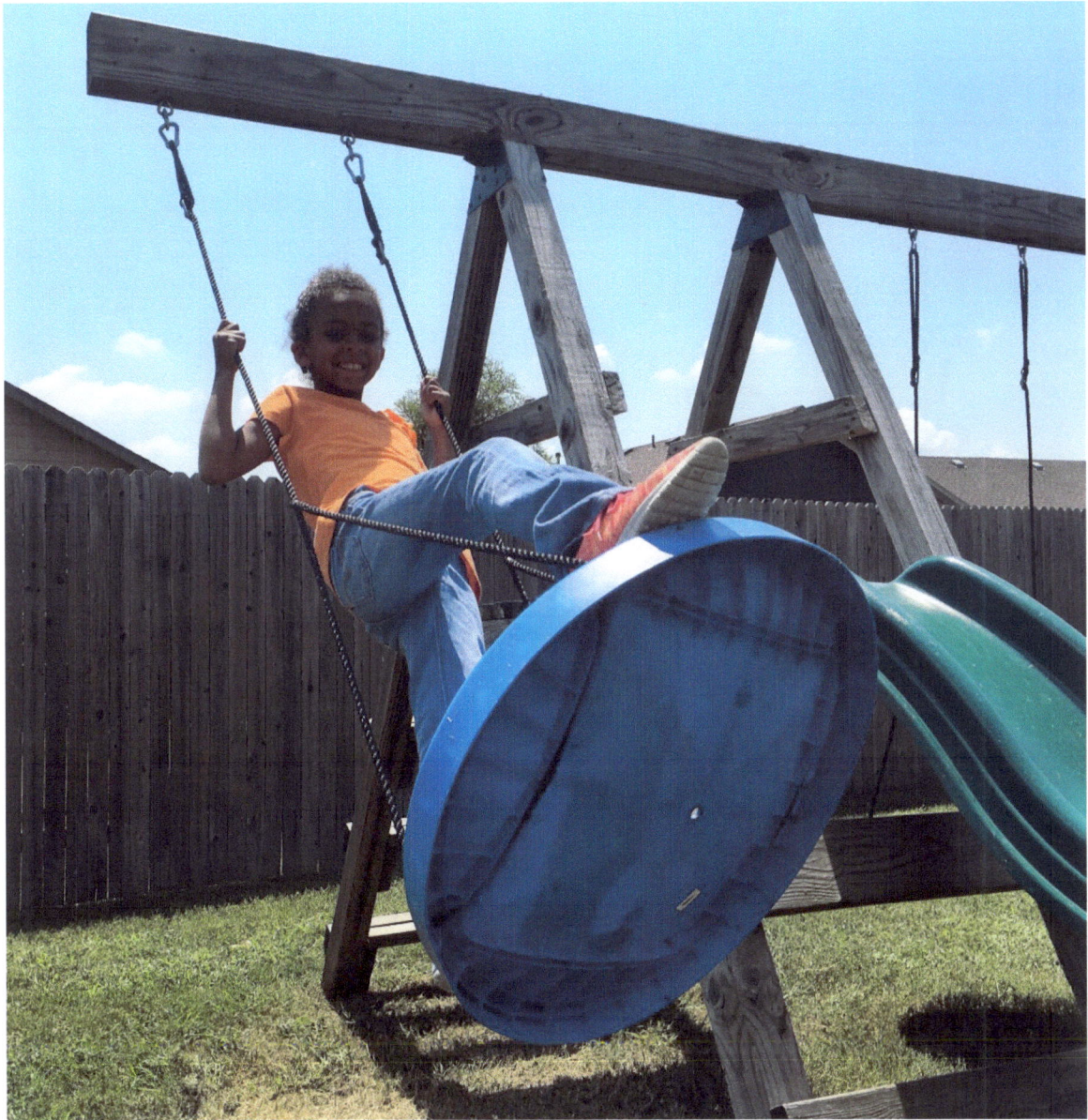

I talk with
my hands.

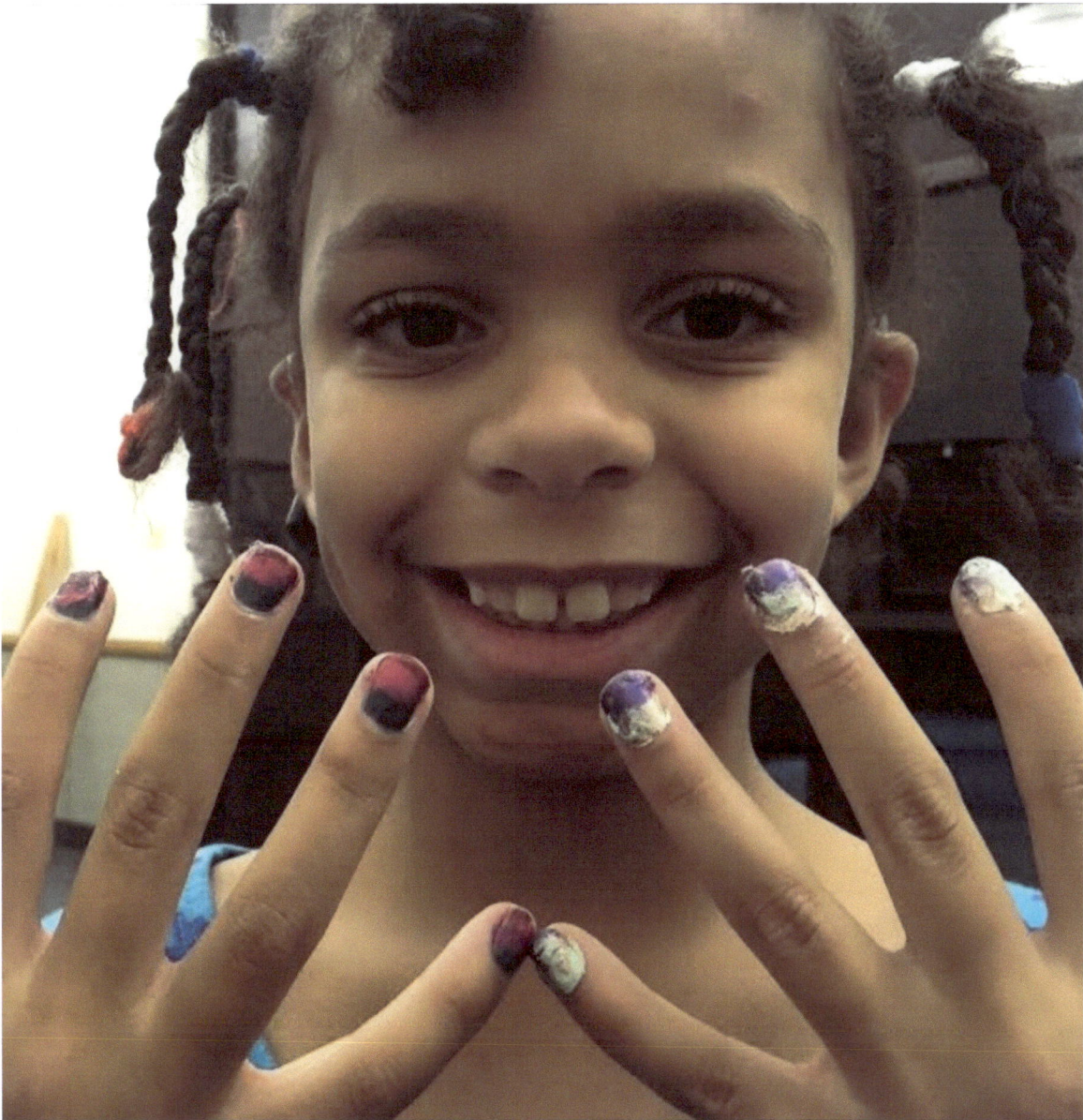

And I sing with my voice.

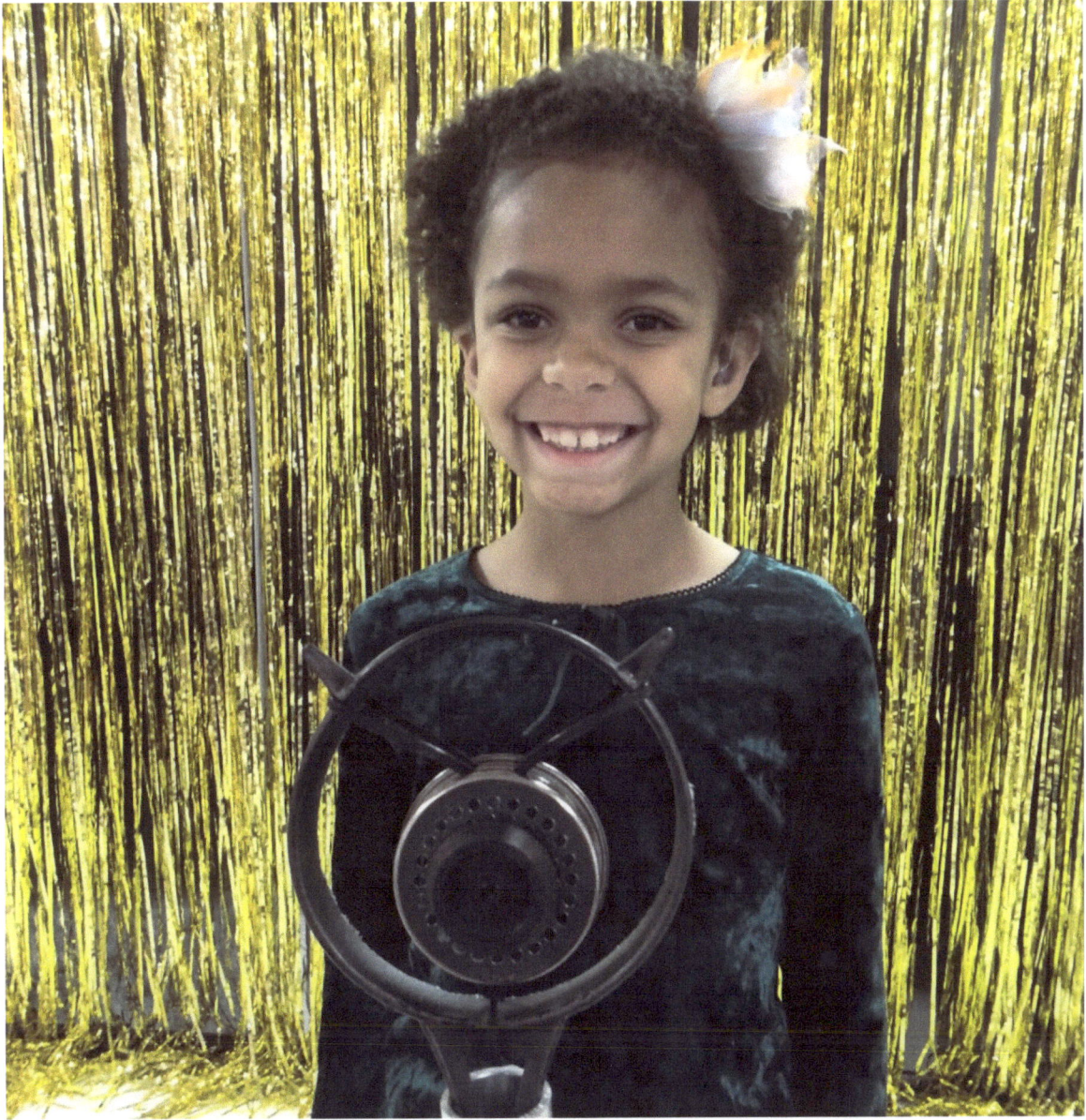

I listen with
my eyes,
and my hands,
and my feet.

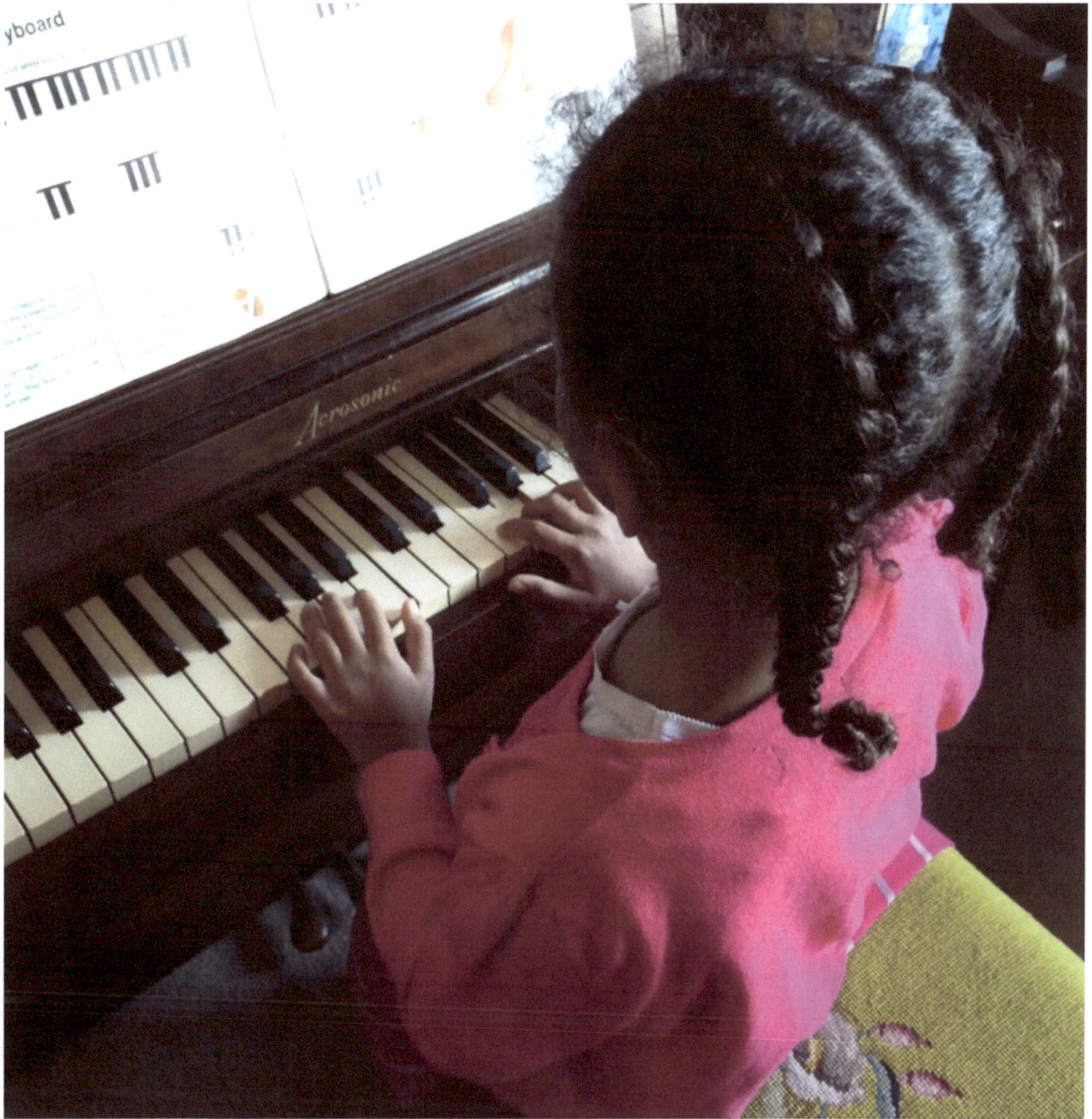

And I listen with tiny computers hidden in my head.

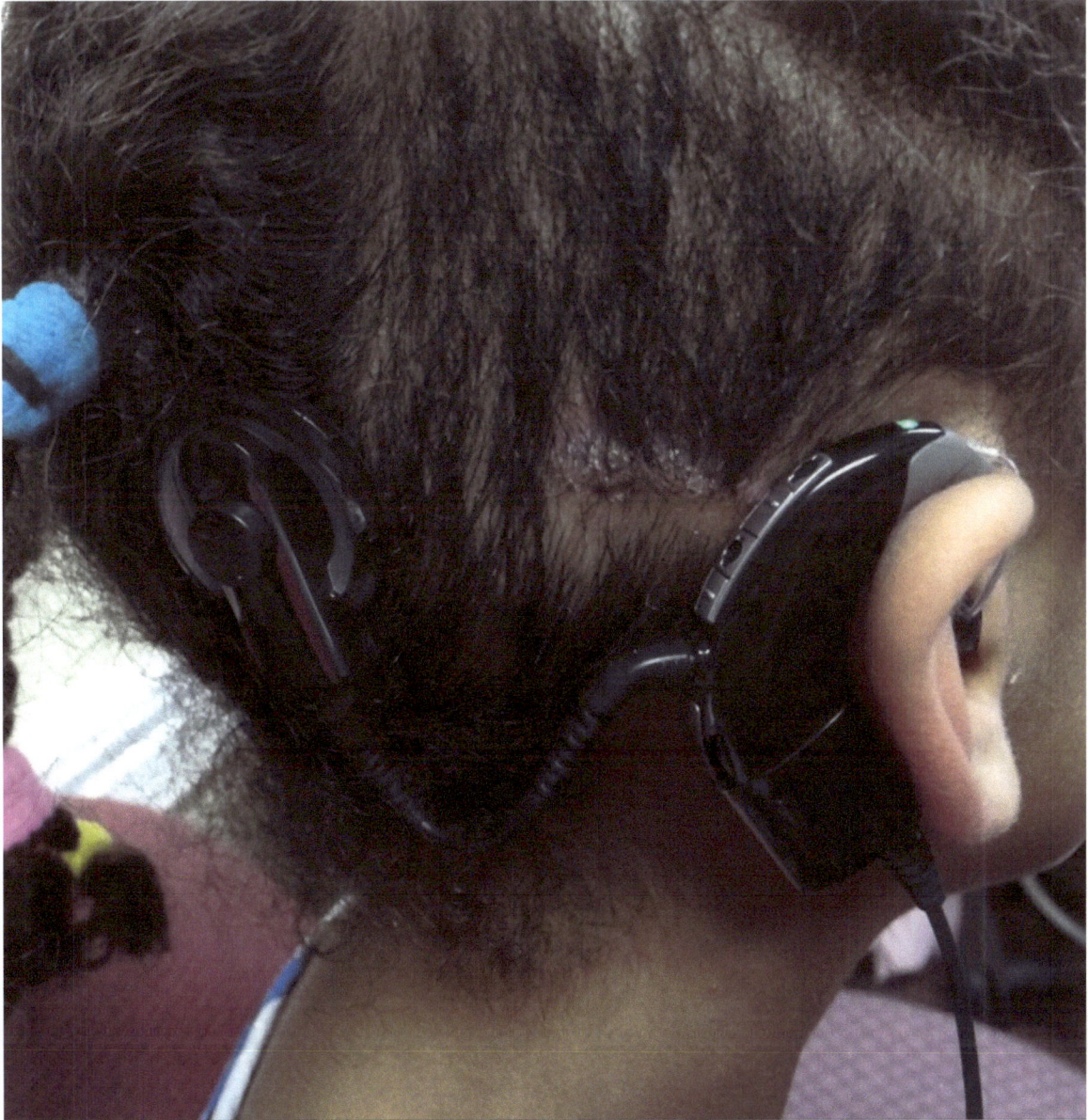

I wasn't
always
this amazing.

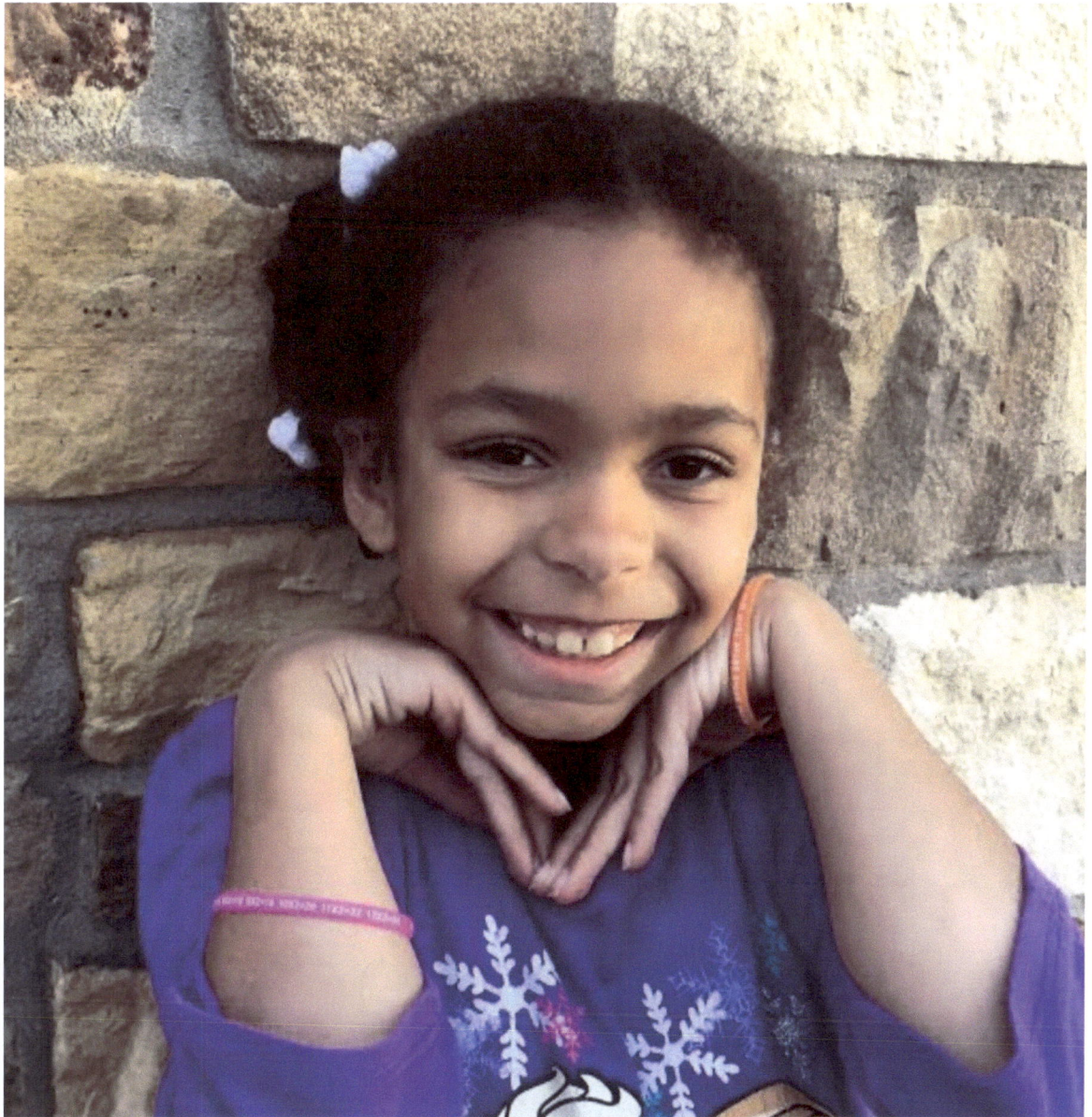

When I was a toddler, my ears stopped working.

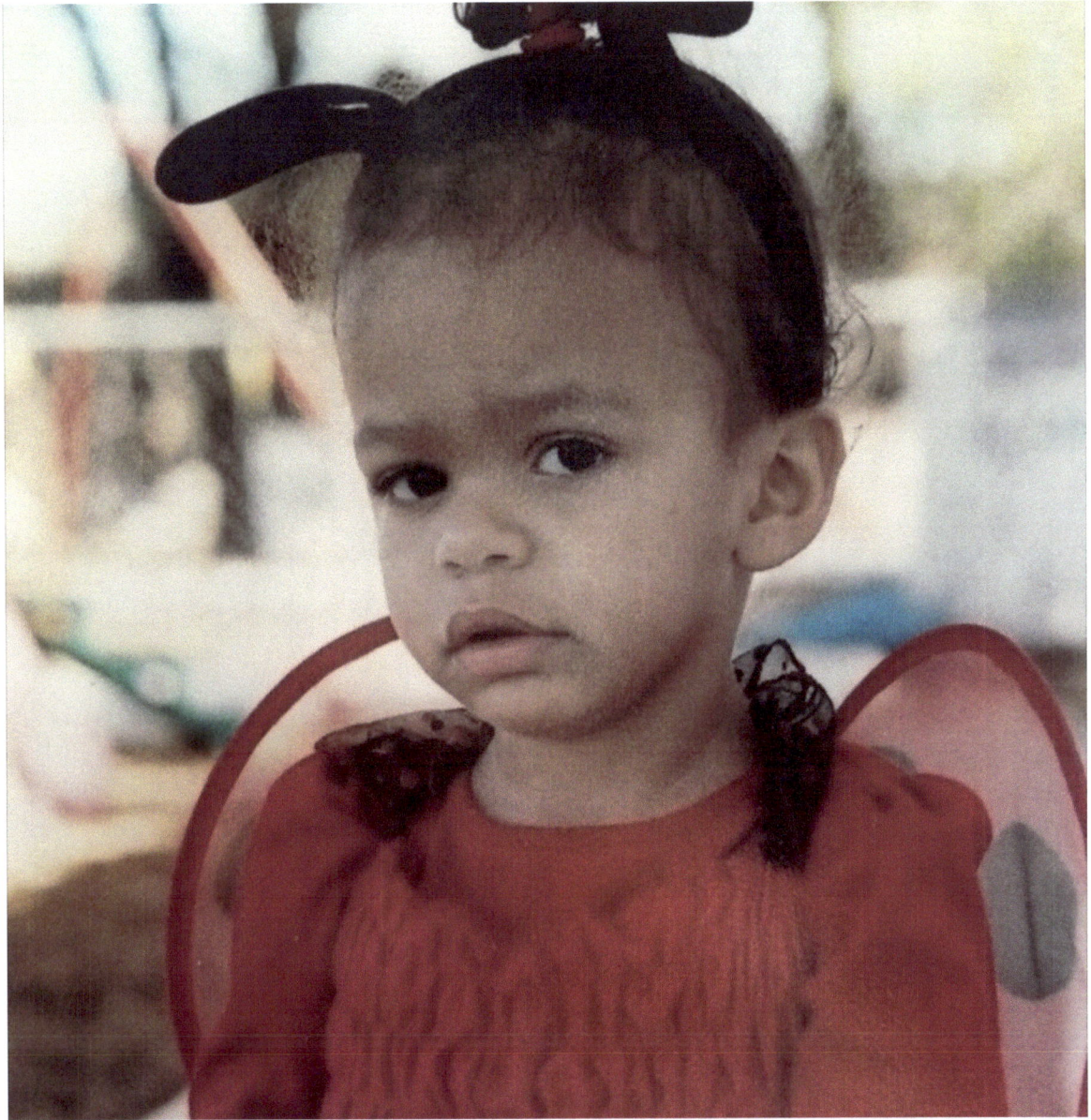

Voices became whispers, and sound went dark.

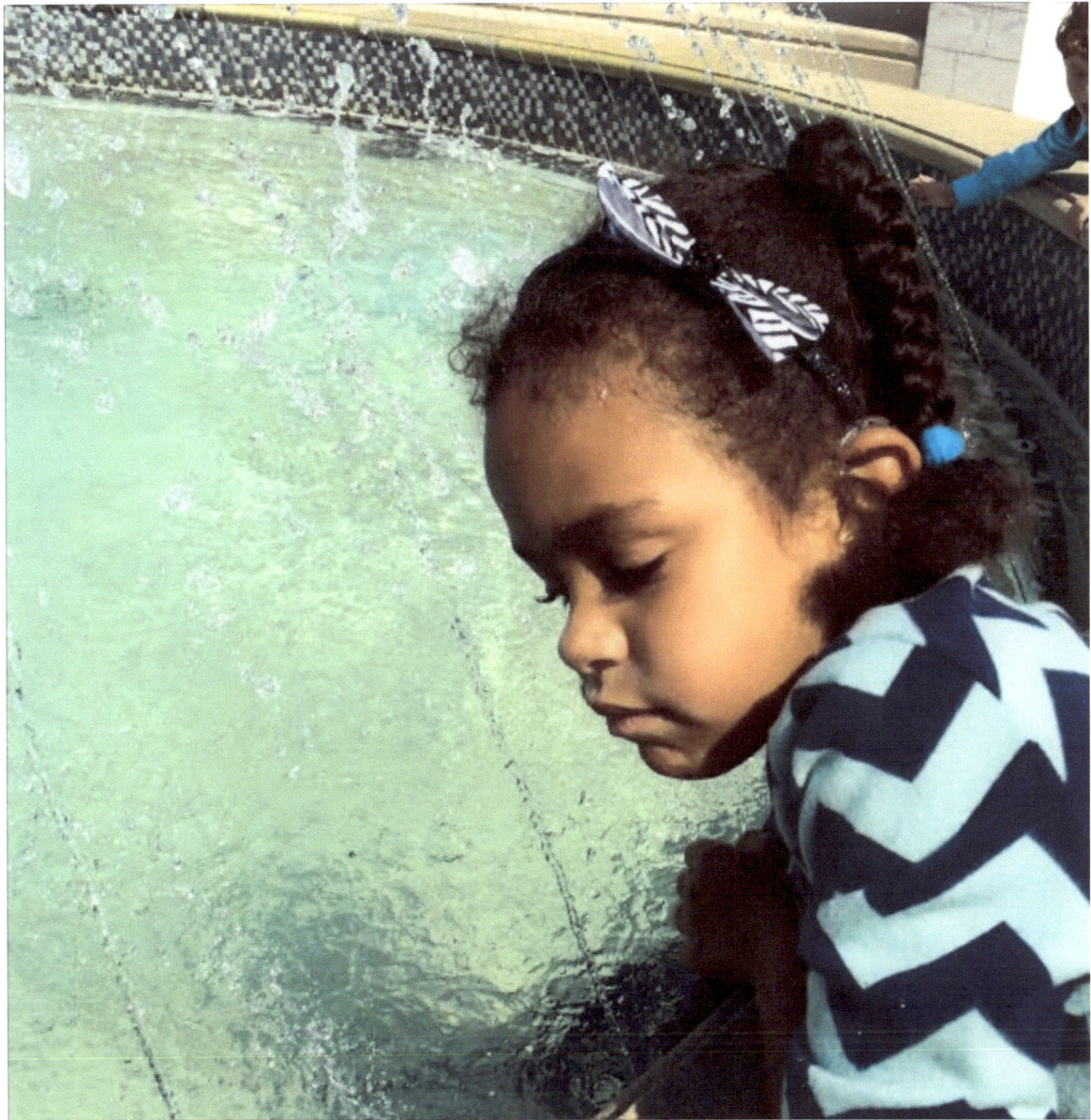

There was so much I I couldn't understand.

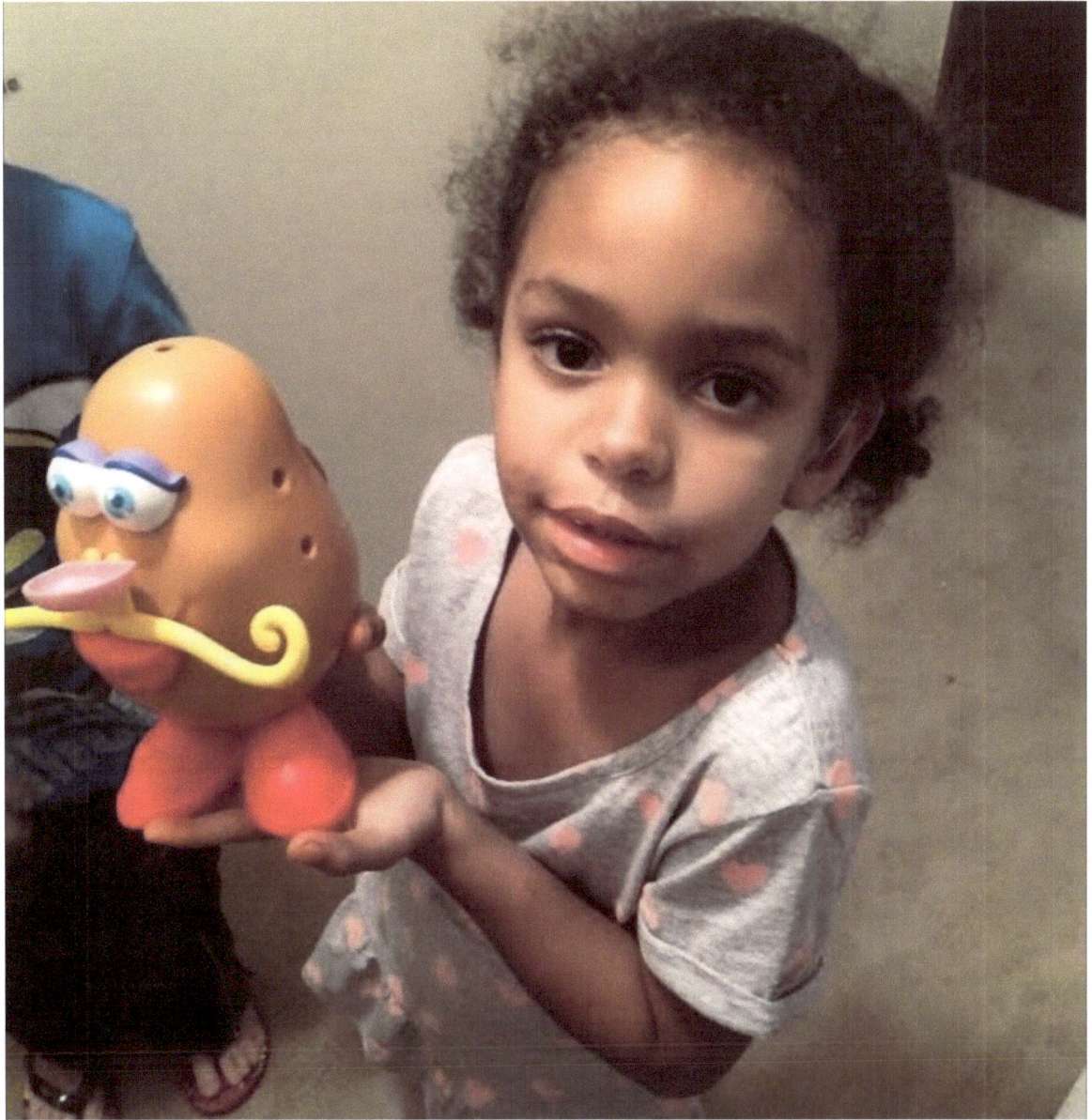

I was all alone, even with everyone around me.

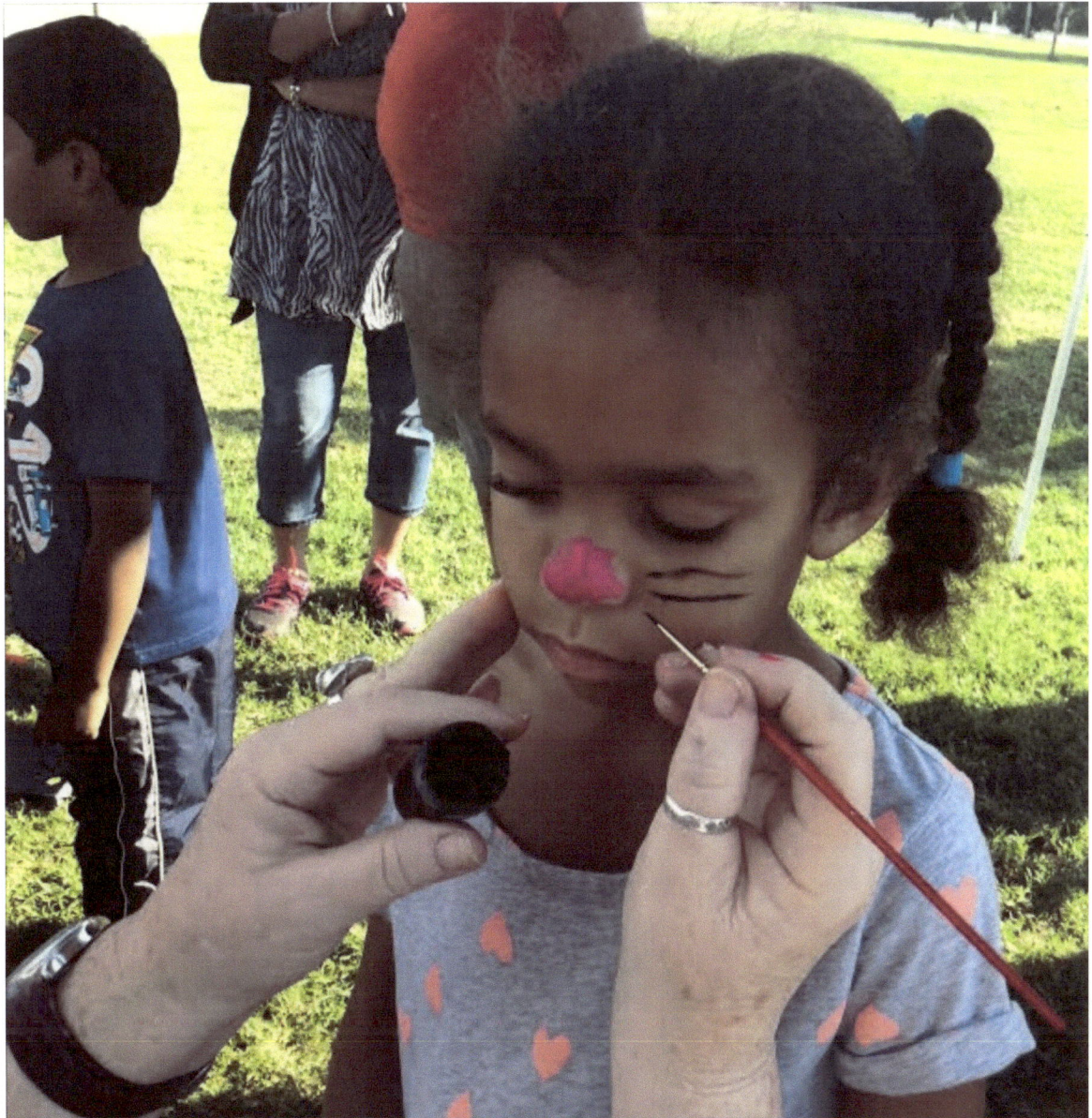

Then, in kindergarten, I started to wear hearing aids.

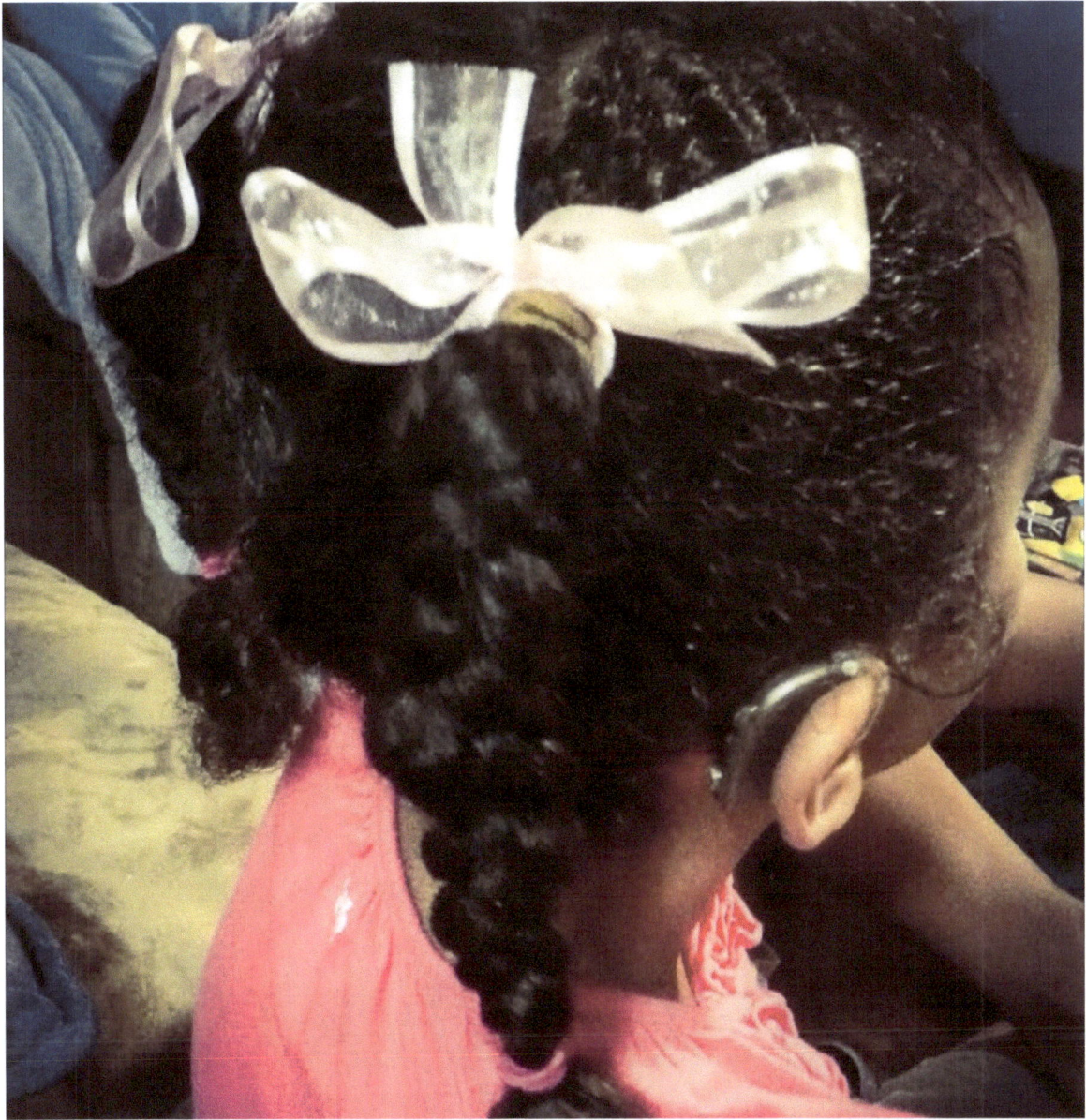

And I found places to help me get better at sign language.

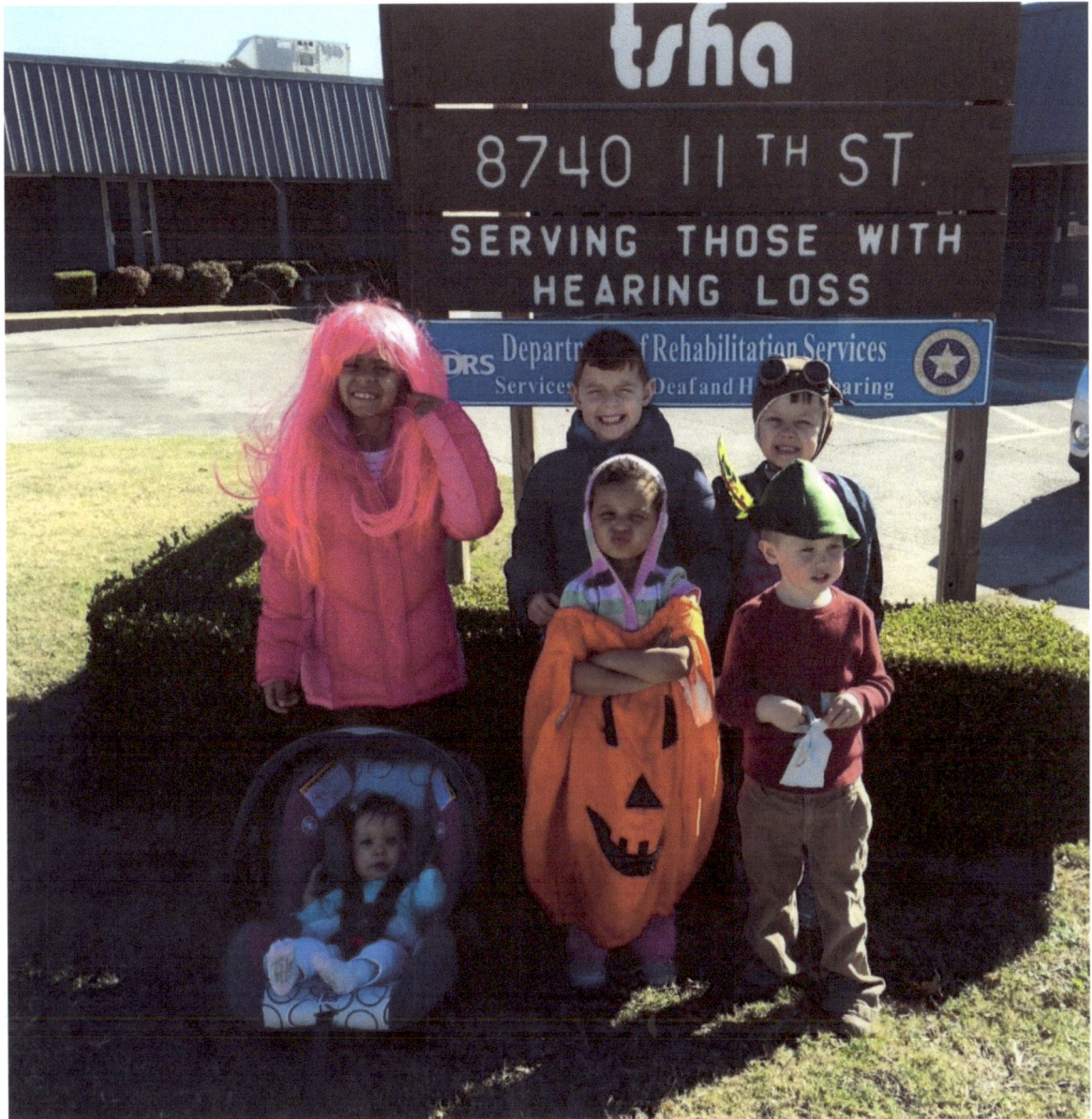

In first grade, I even got to go to Deaf school!

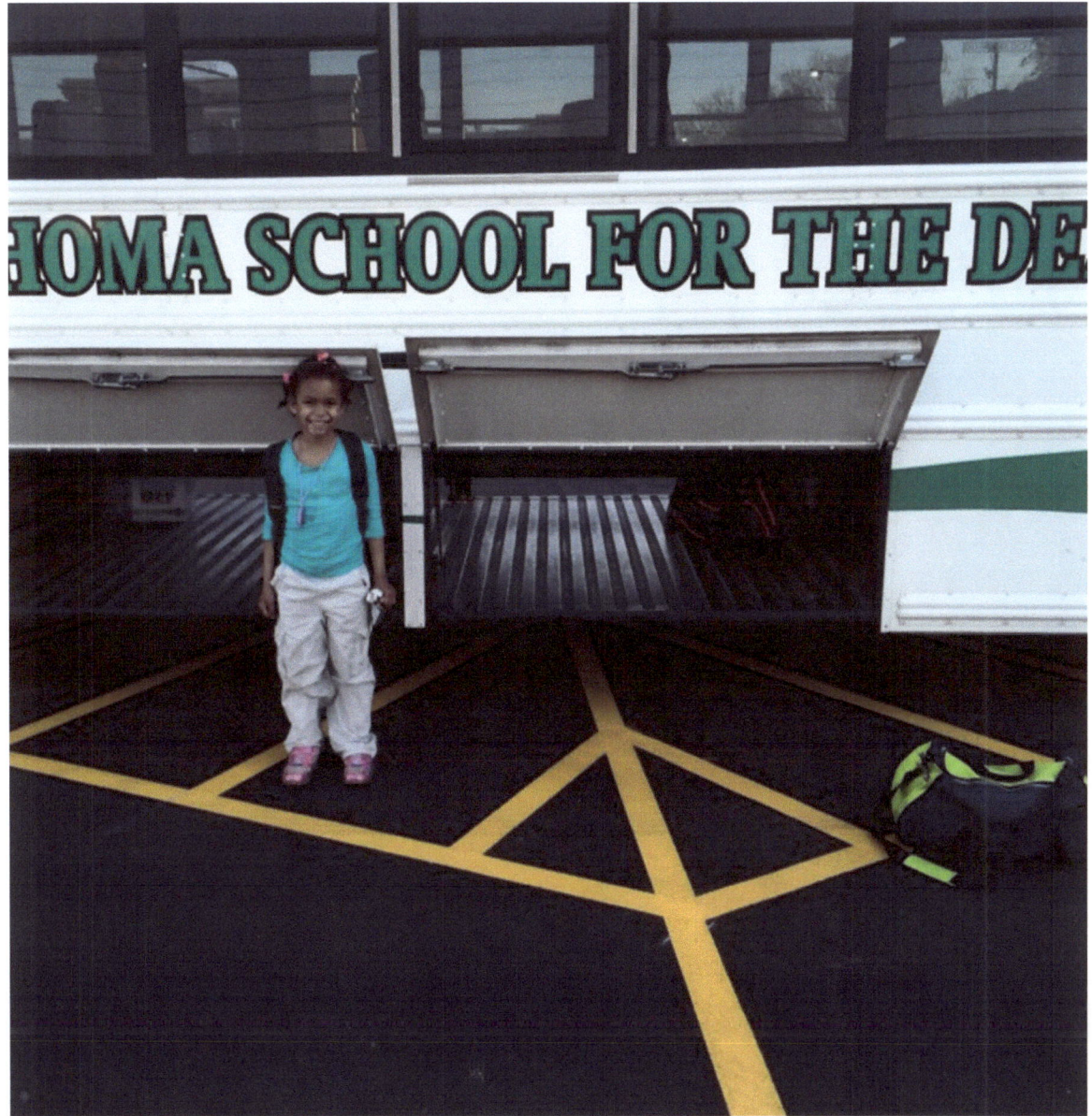

Sometimes hearing aids and sign language made life marvelous!

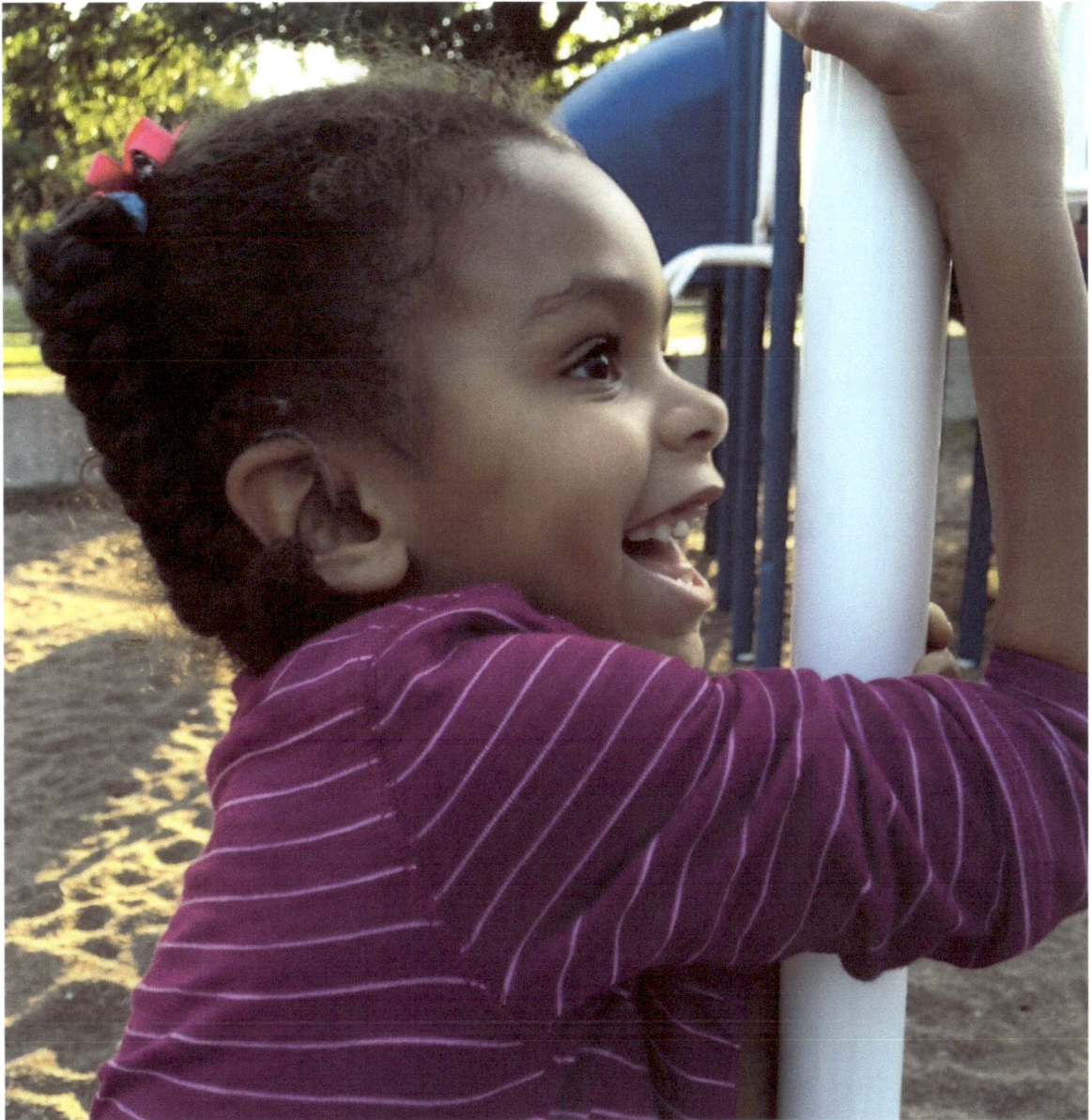

Sometimes it wasn't enough.

I still felt left out.

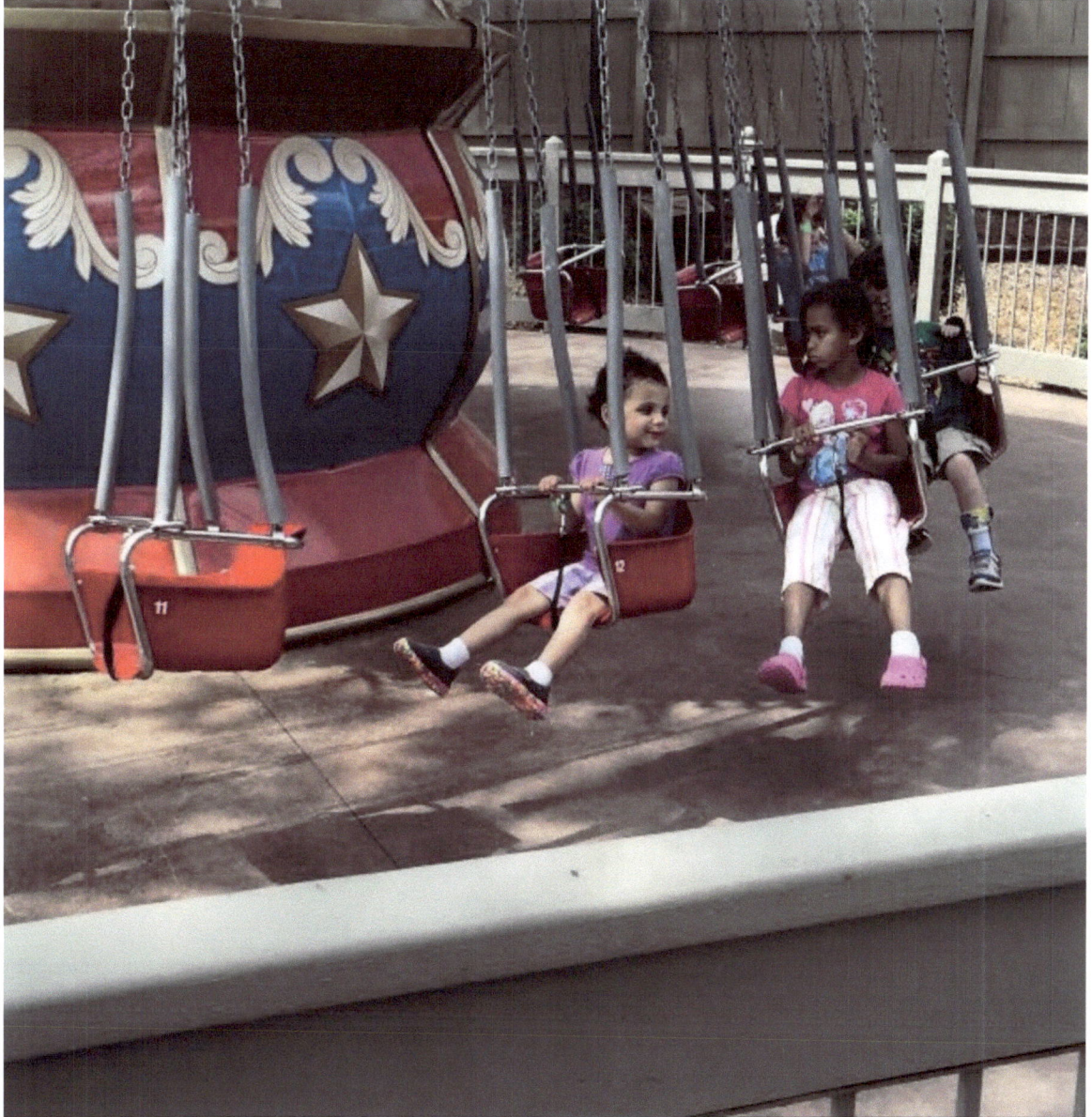

I told my
ear doctor
I wanted to
understand
even more.

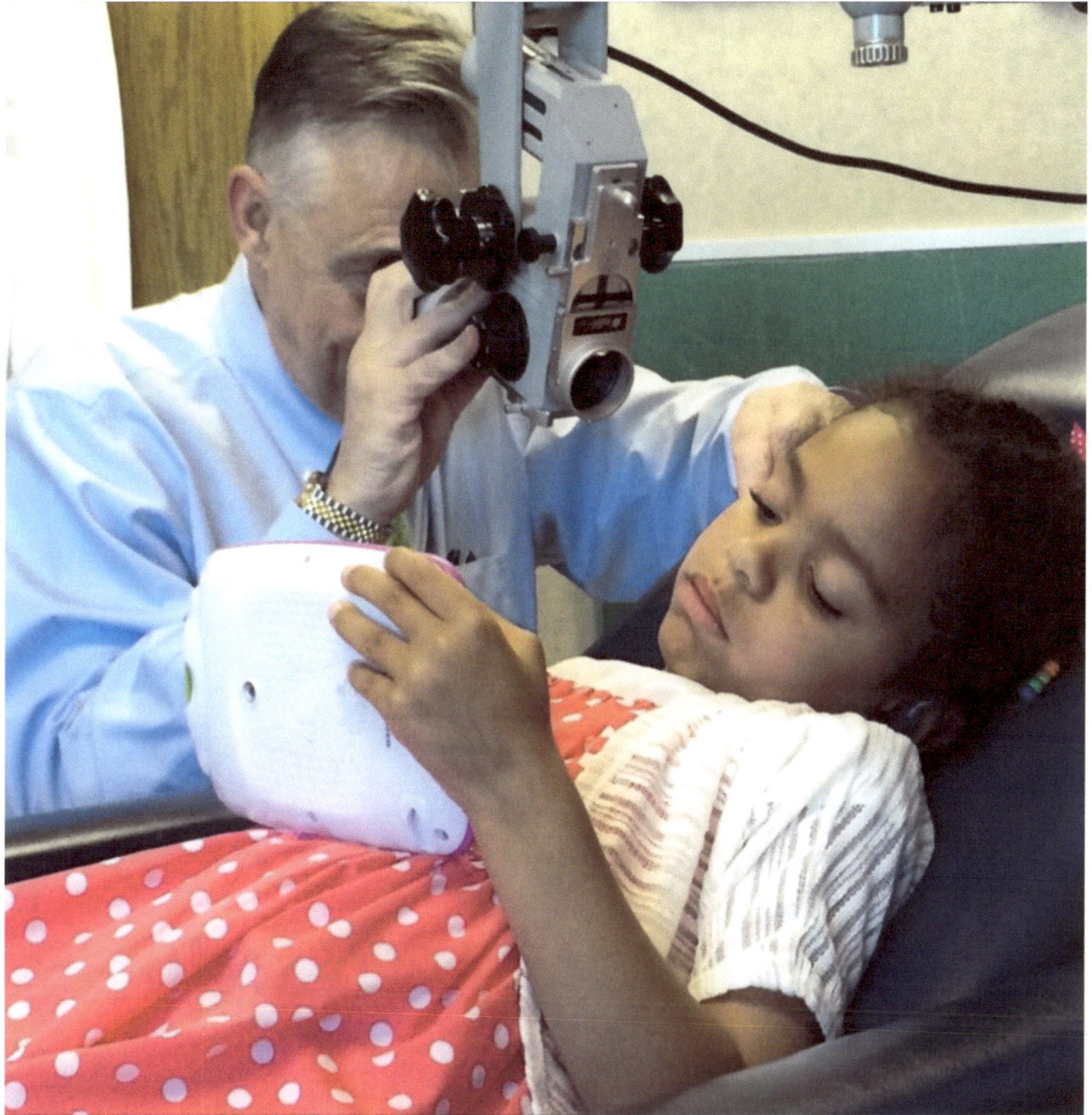

I chose to get cochlear implants.

(That meant going to the hospital to have surgery on my head!)

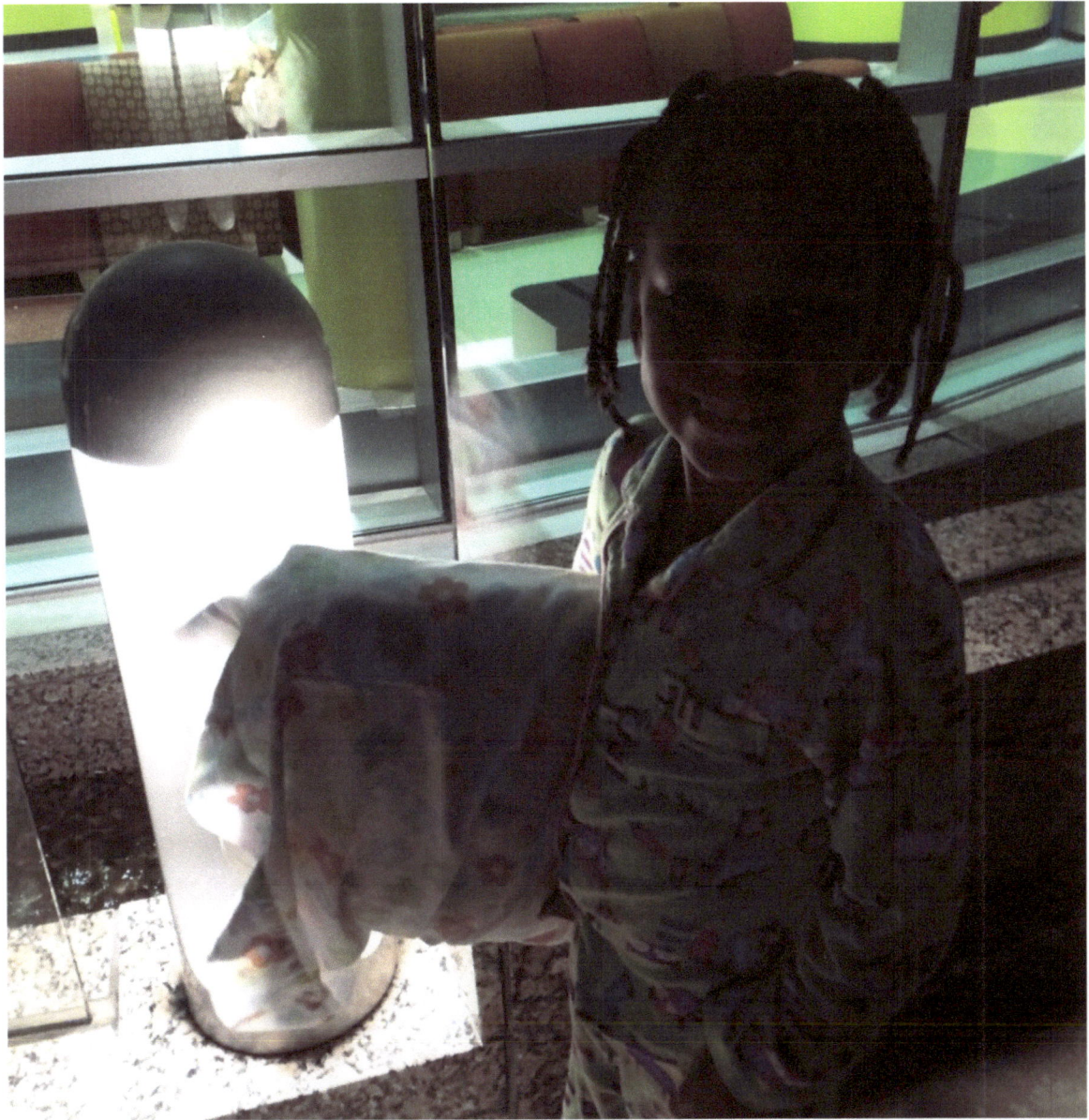

It was very early in the morning, and I felt a little nervous.

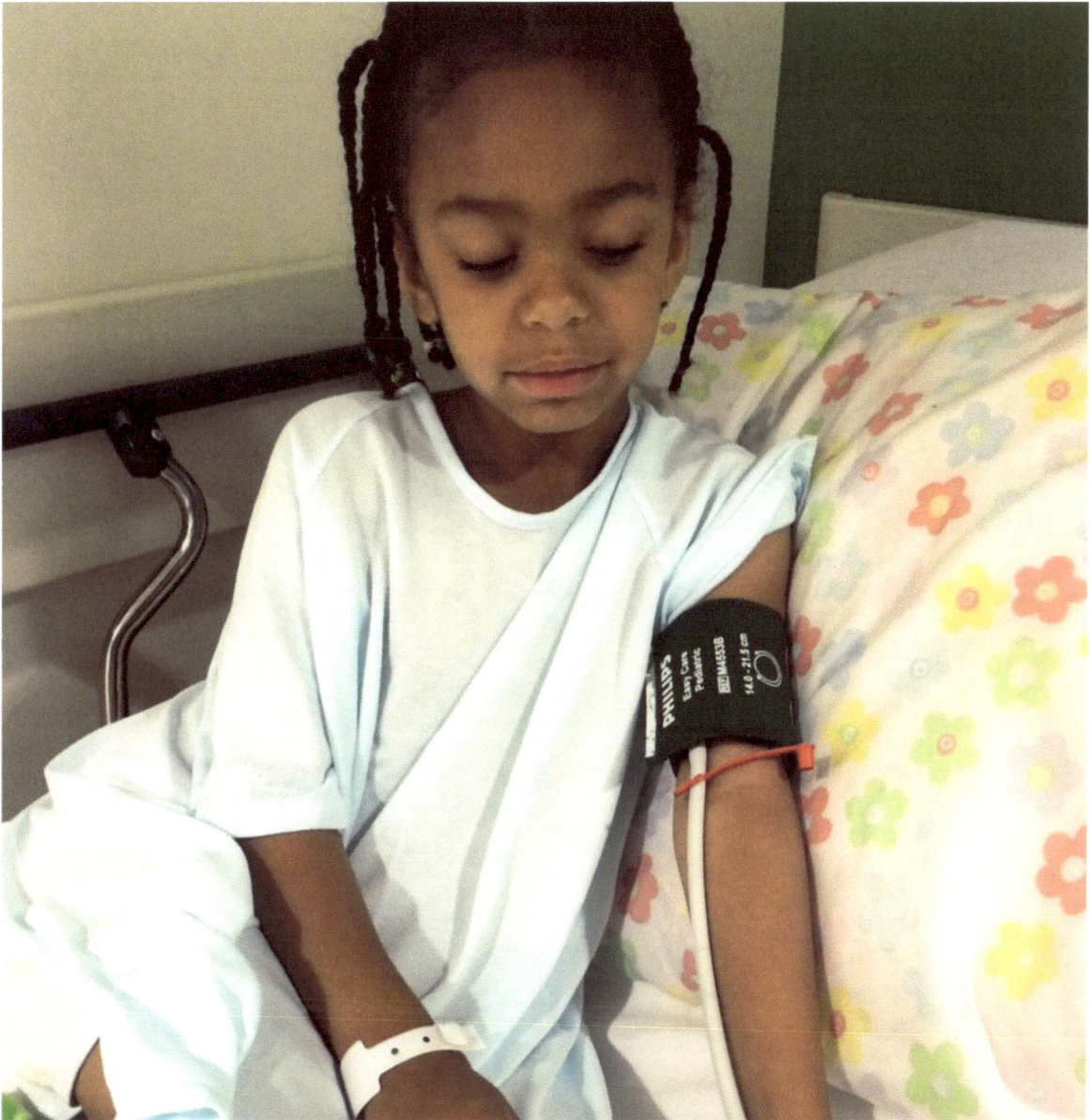

They gave me
some sleepy
medicine, and
then rolled
me away
to surgery.

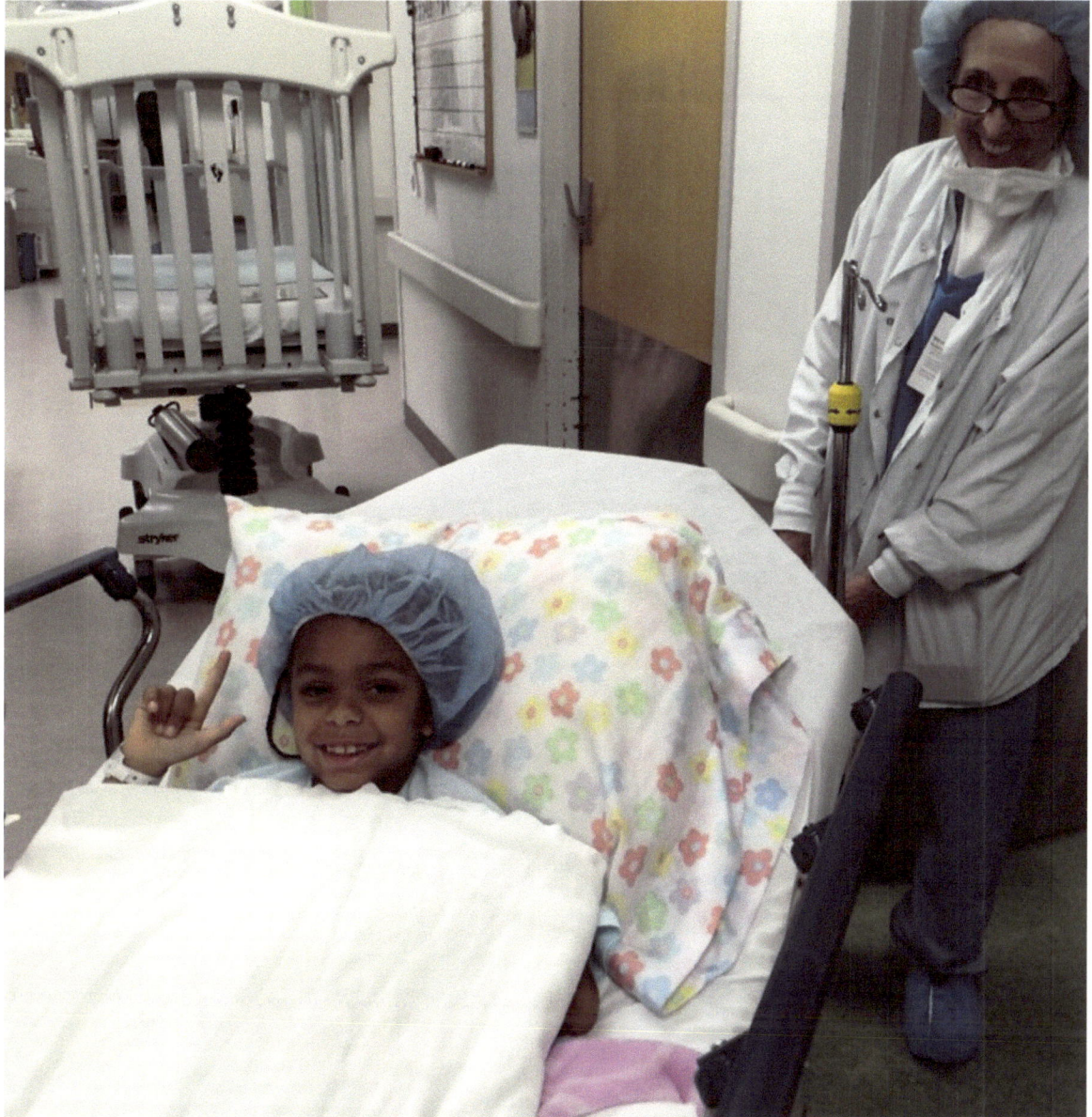

When I woke up after surgery, my head sure did hurt!

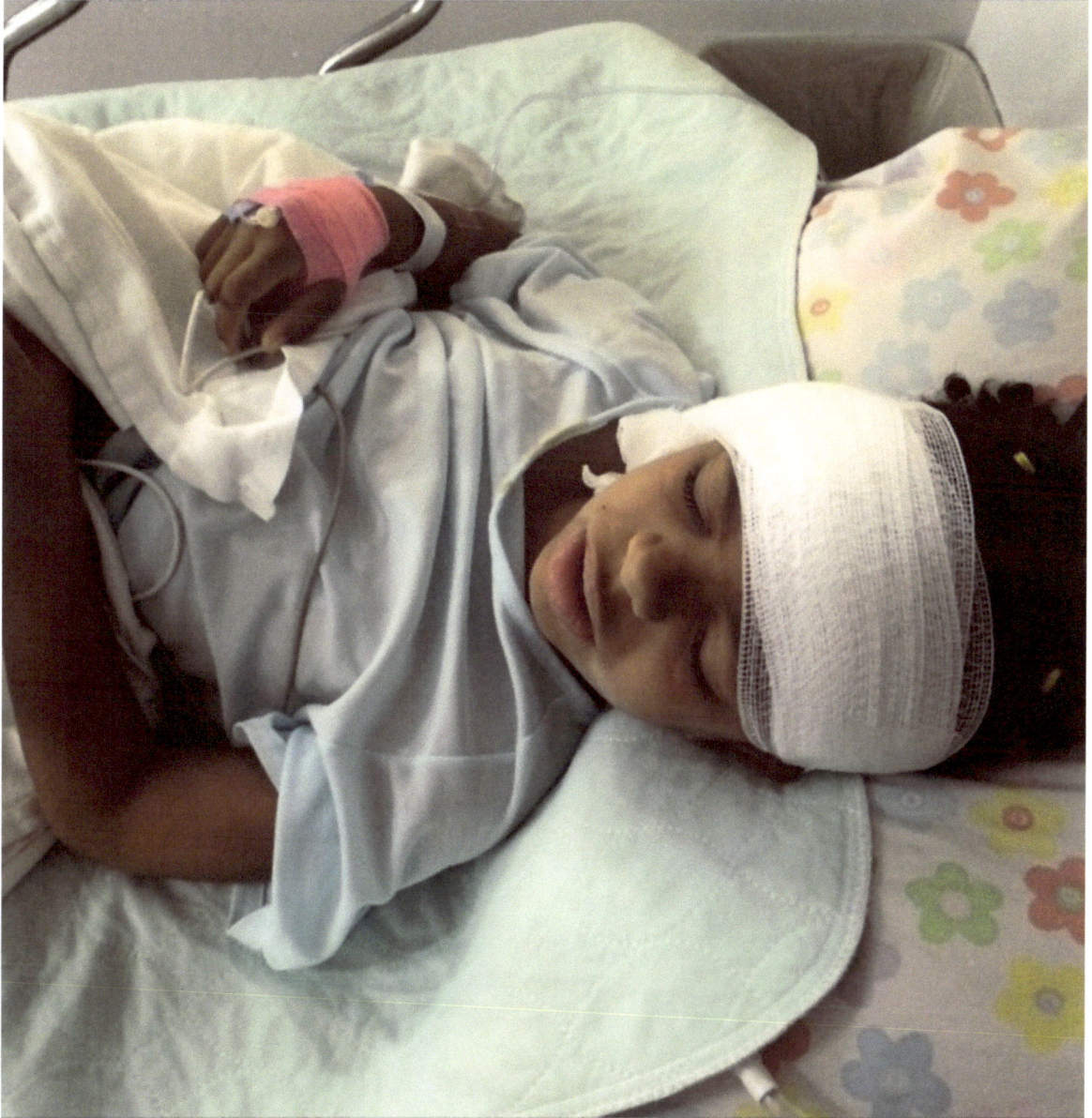

I slept all the way home.

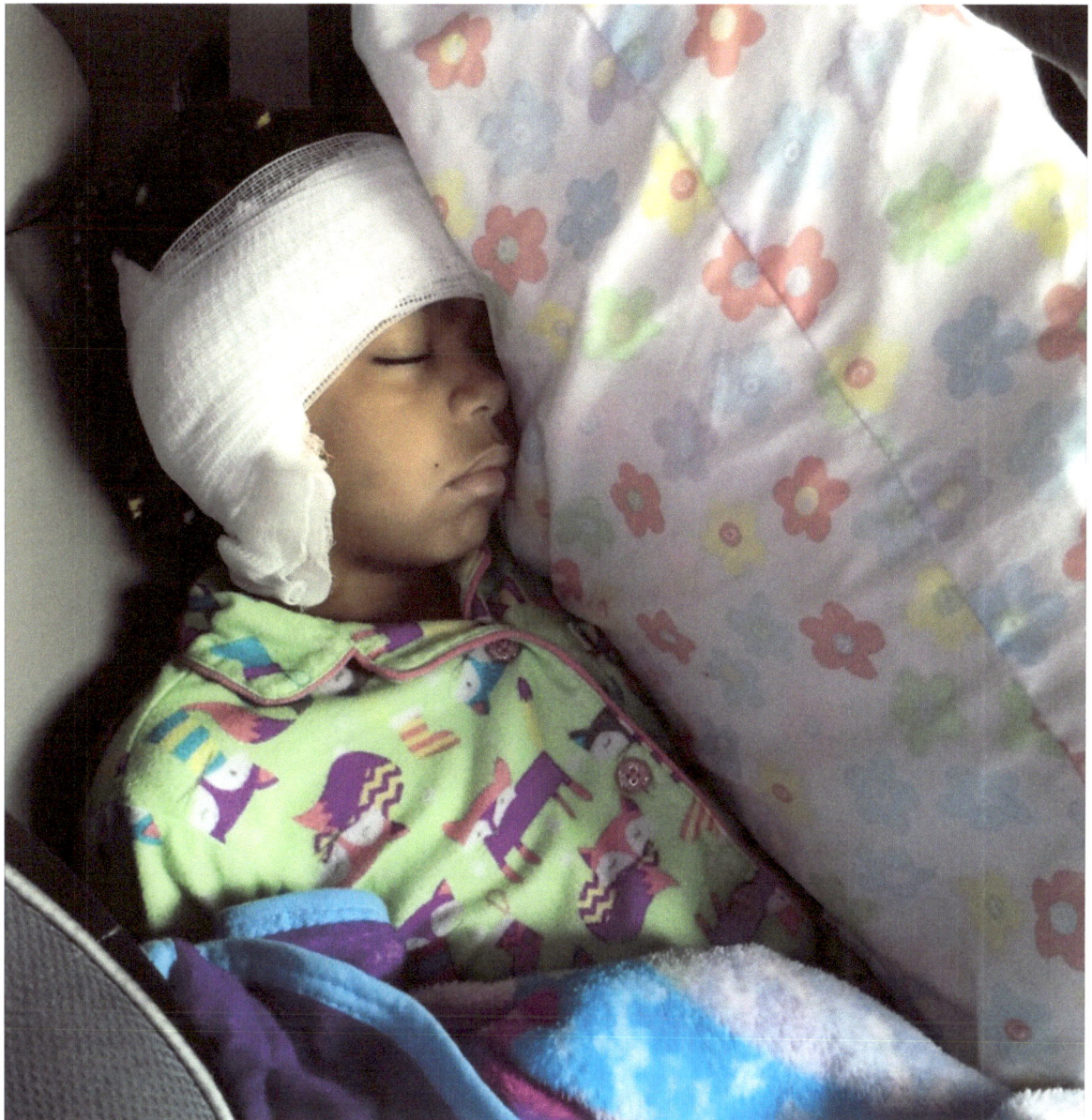

But I felt better the next morning!

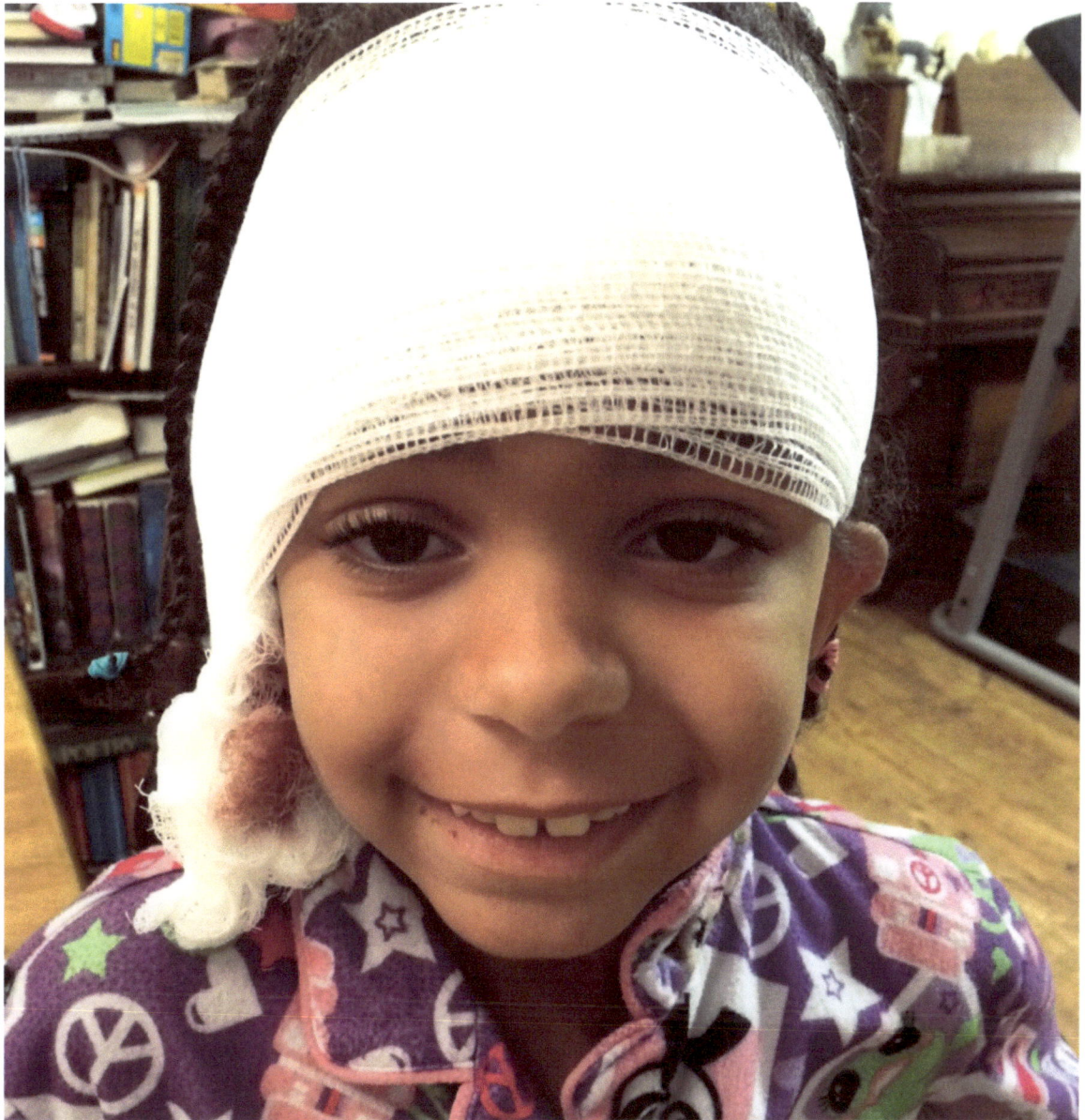

I couldn't wait for my bandages to come off.

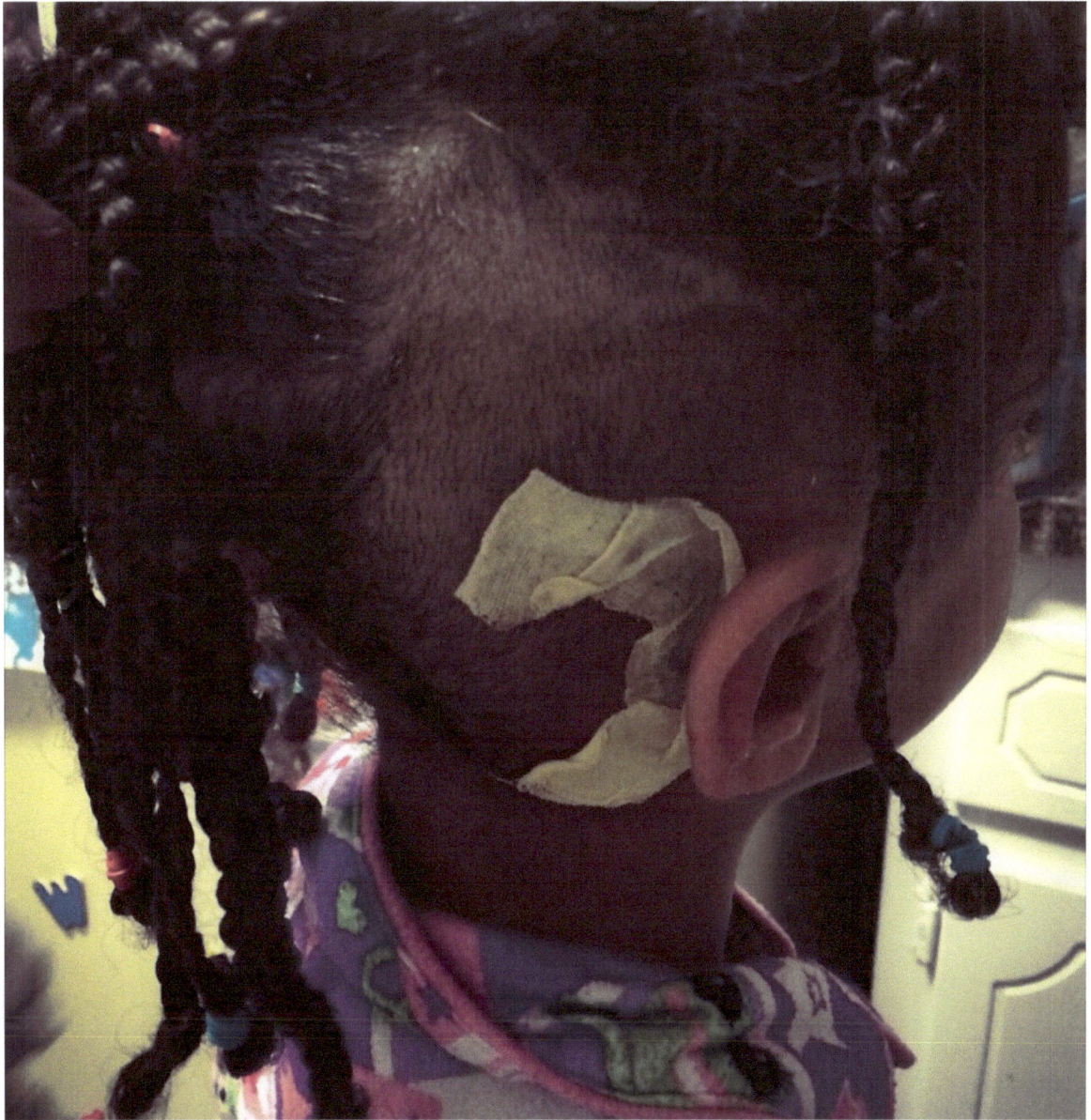

A few weeks later, my audiologist gave me the outside part of my implant.

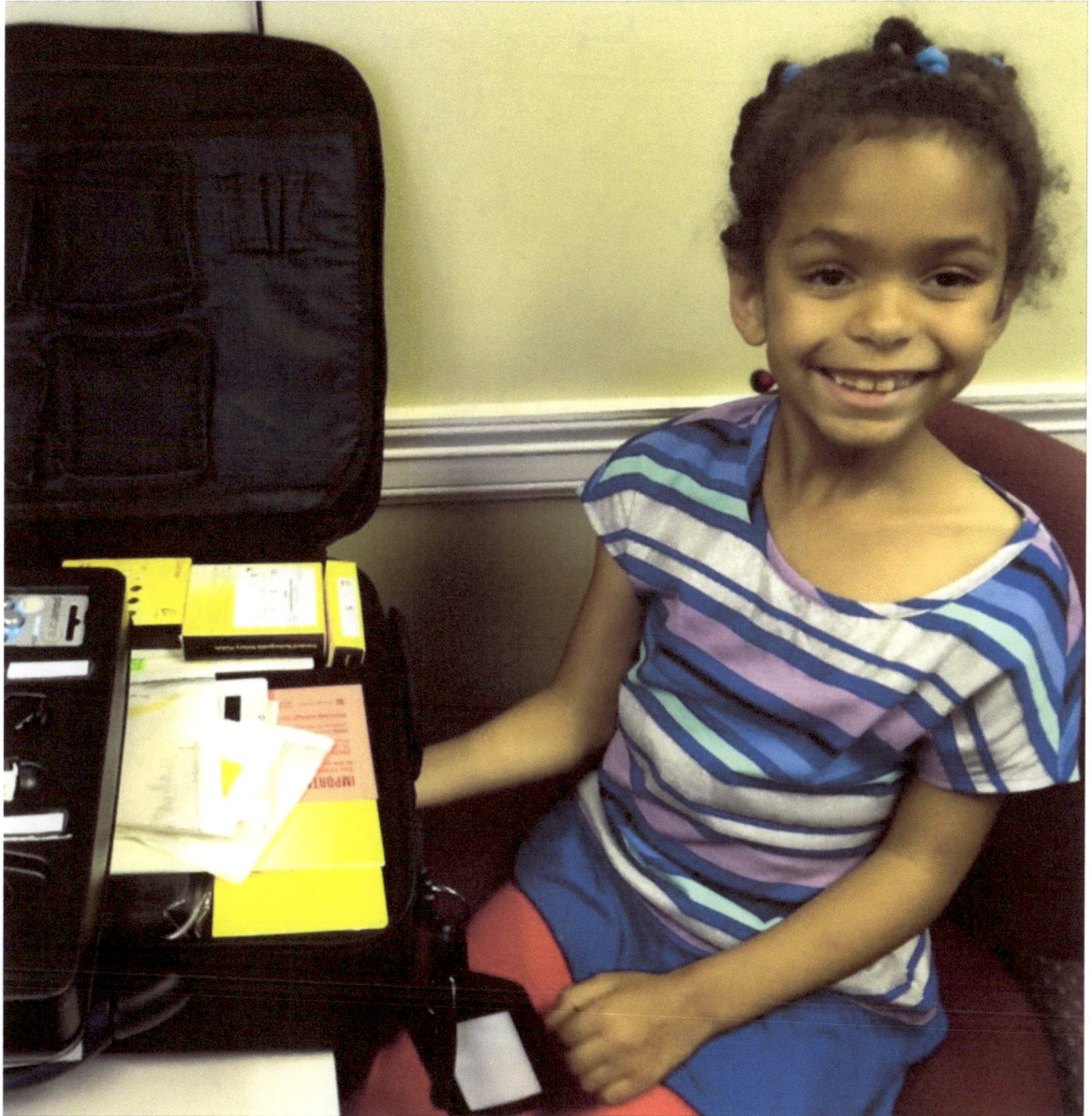

She turned on the processor, and made sure it was working right.

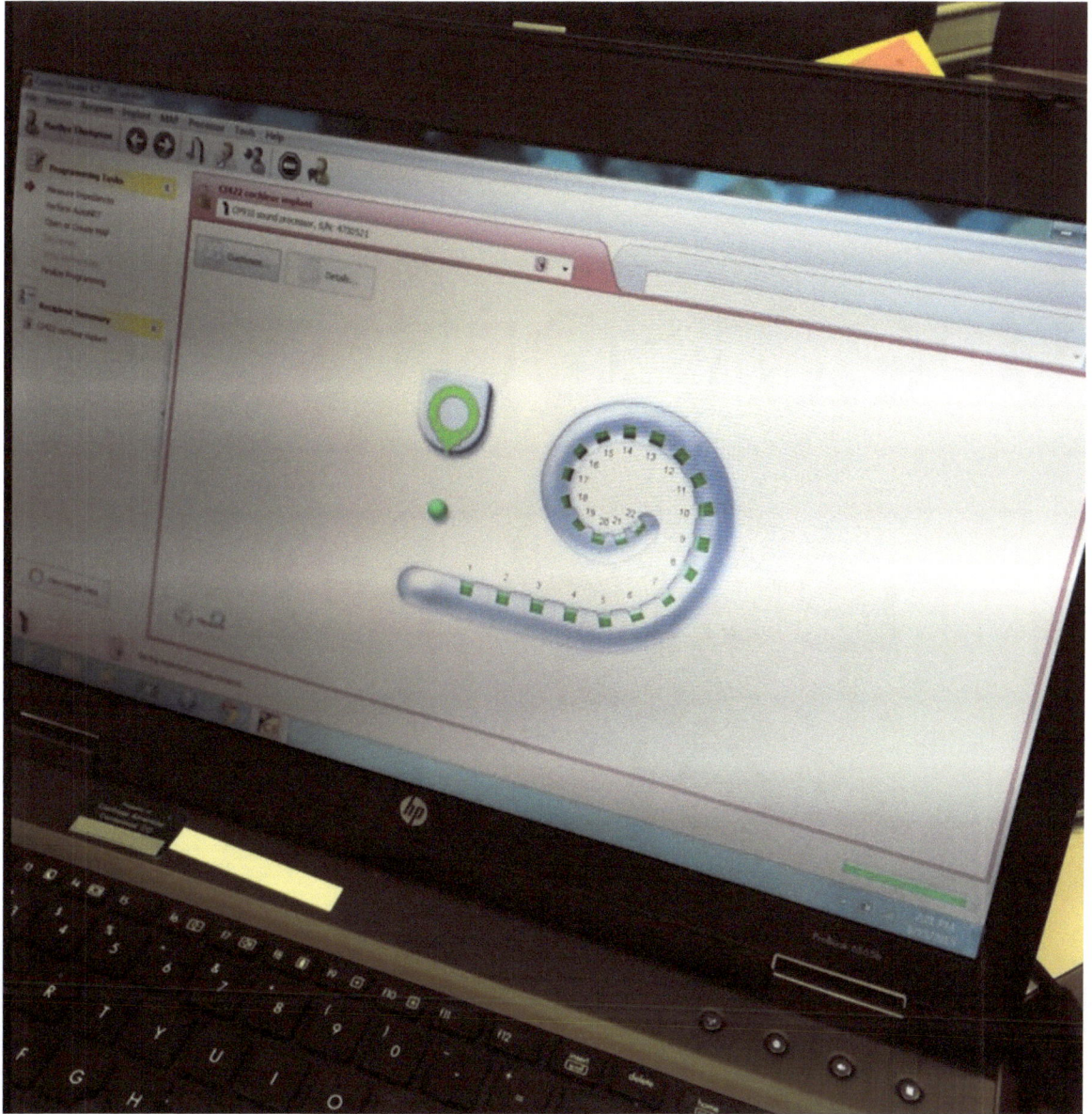

When I
went outside,

I heard birds
for the
first time.

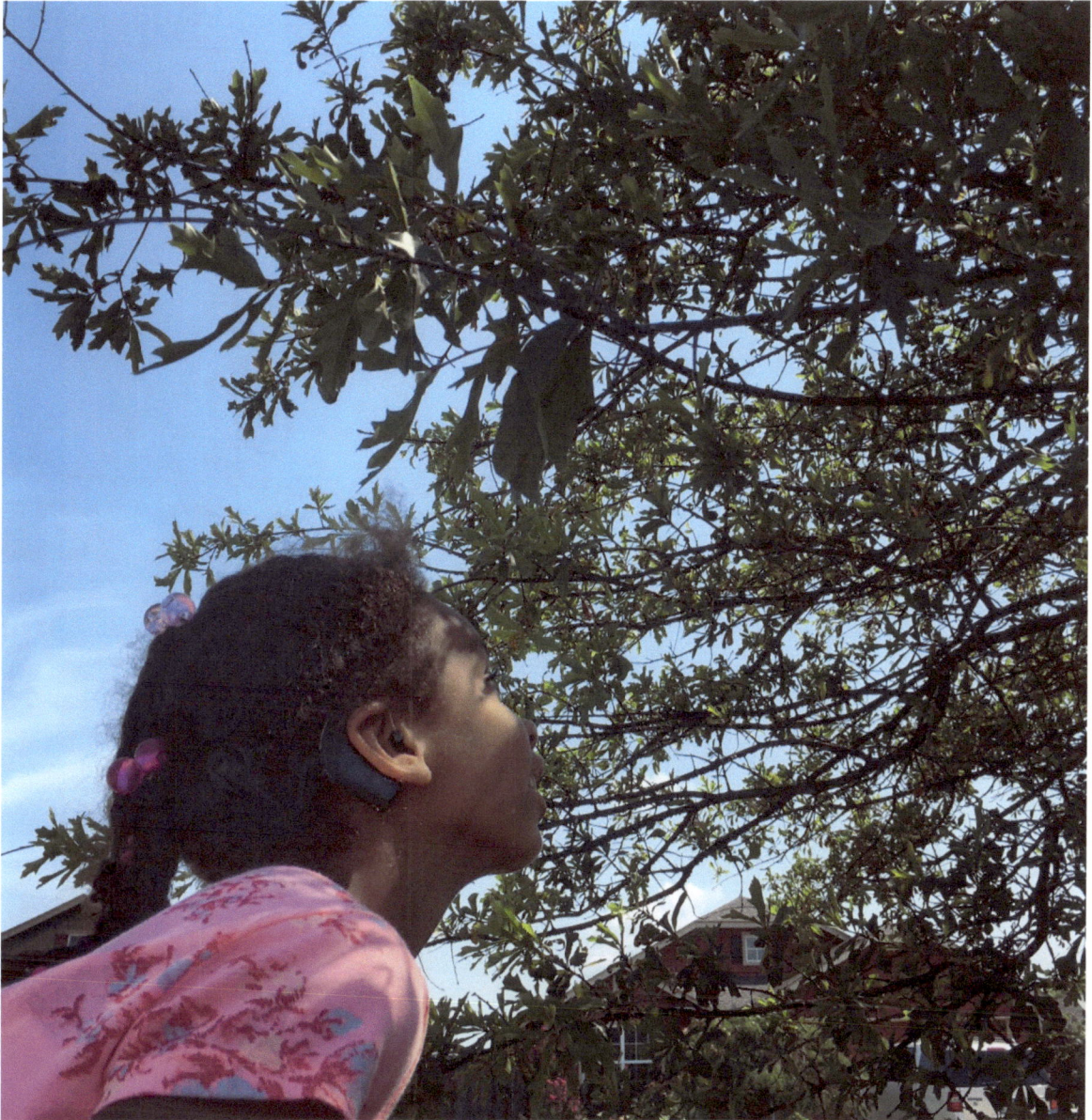

I love my cochlear implants!

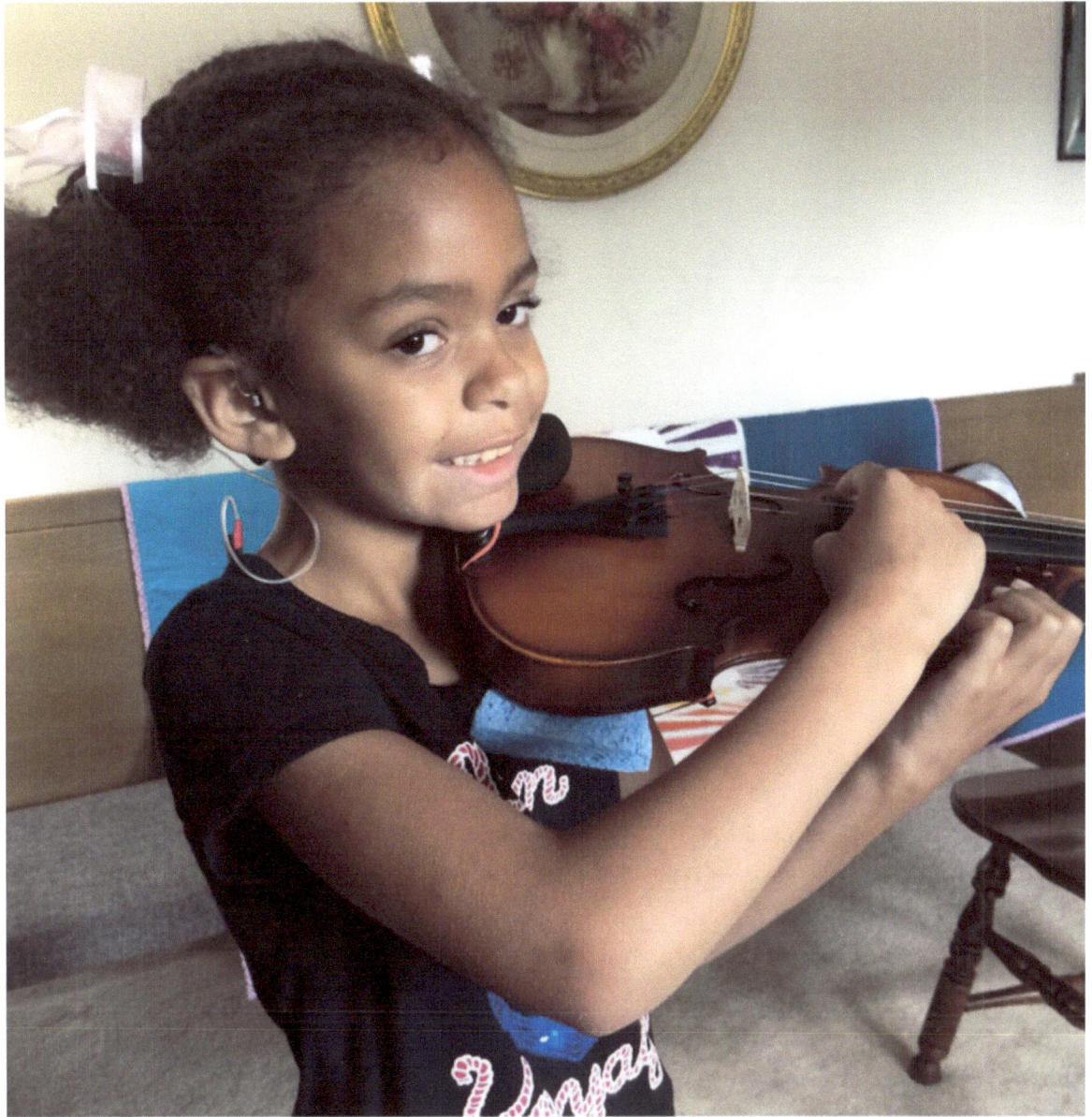

And I still love talking with my hands!

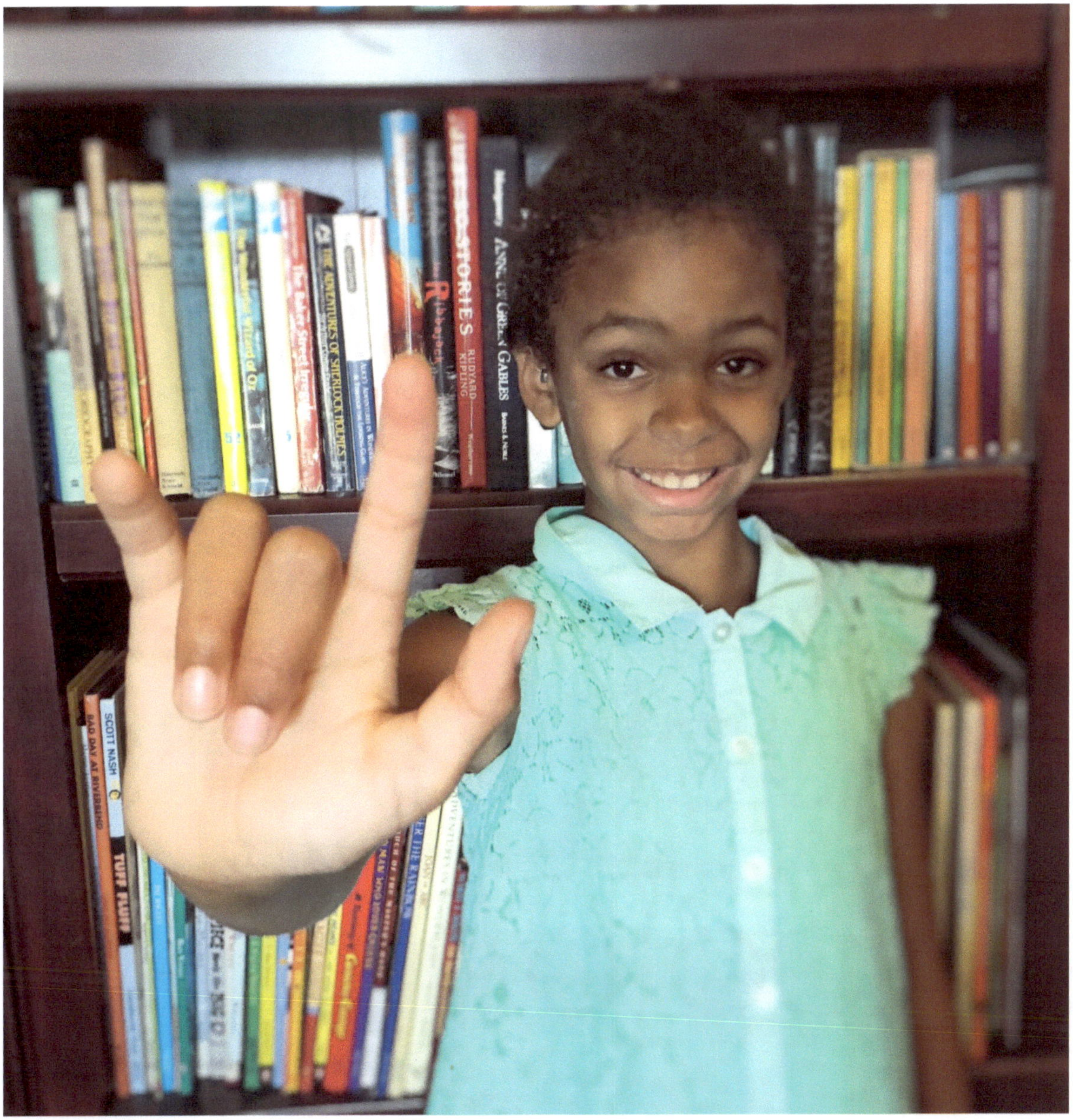
STORIES
RUDYARD KIPLING
ANNE OF GREEN GABLES
THE ADVENTURES OF SHERLOCK HOLMES
SCOTT NASH
TUFF FLUFF
BAD DAY AT RIVERBEND

With both together, my life is so much more colorful!

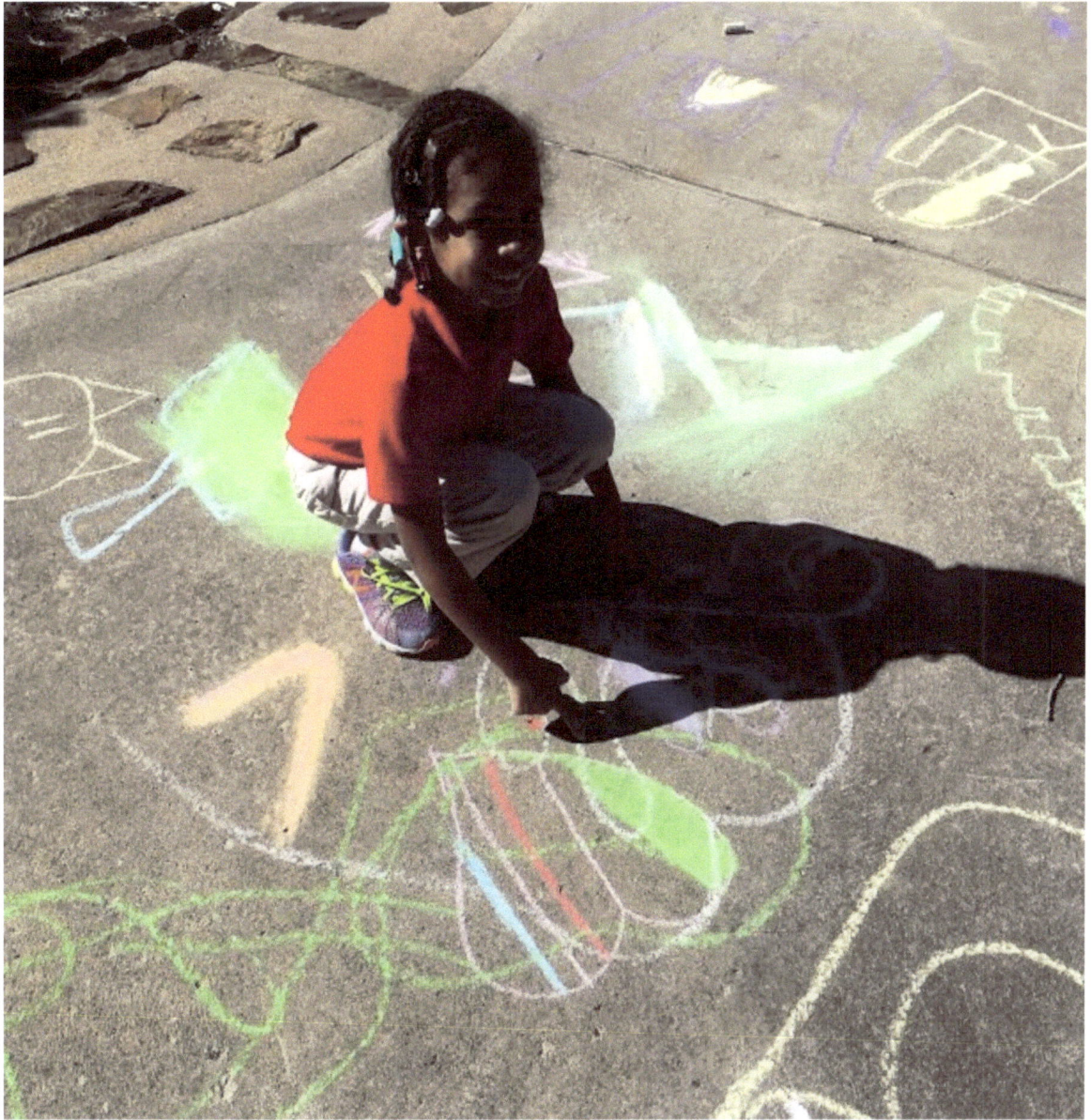

And that's absolutely marvelous.

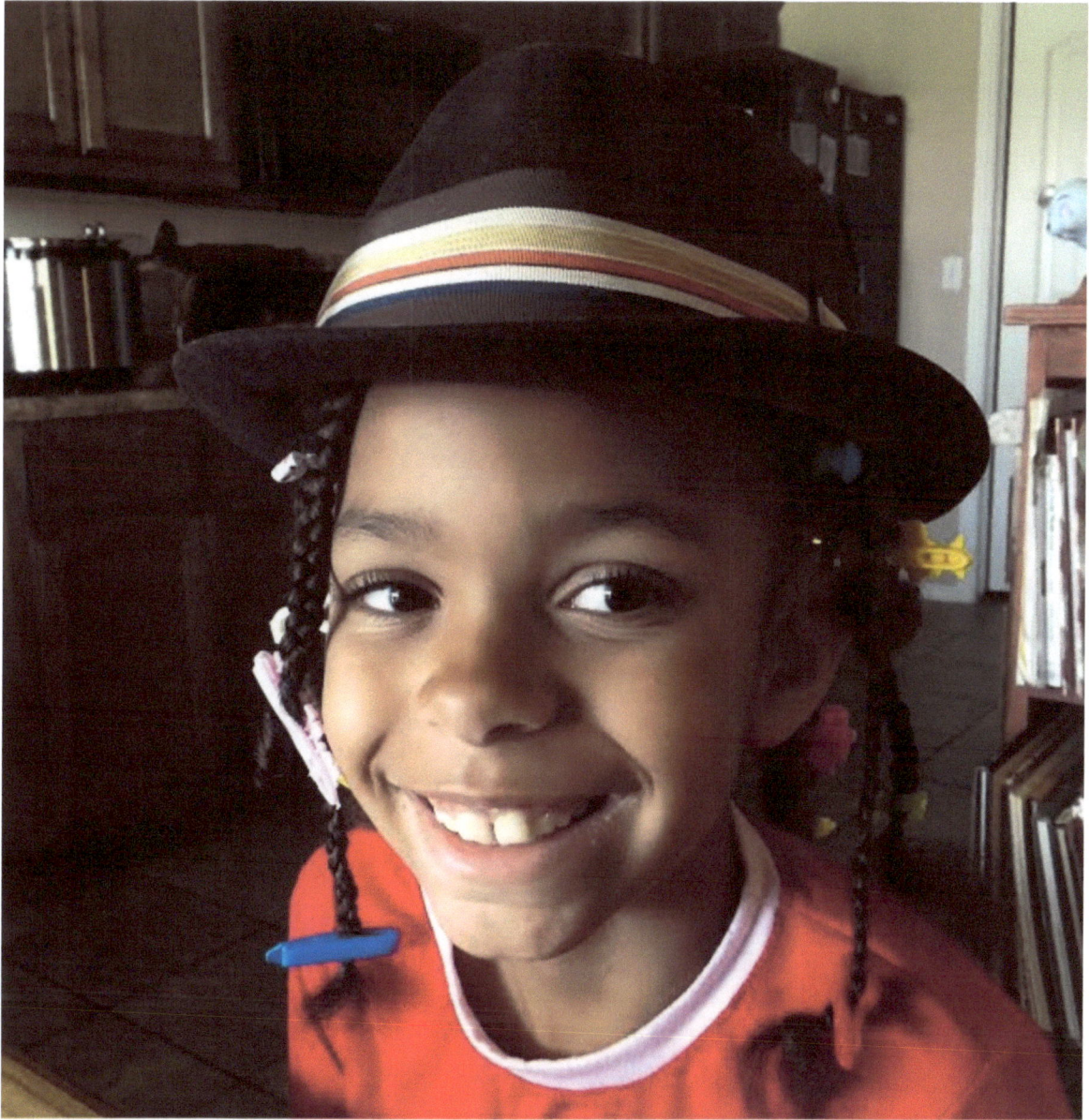

First Printing: 2017

ISBN: 978-0-9977588-7-0

HWC Press, LLC
P.O. Box 3792
Bartlesville, OK 74006

housewifeclass@gmail.com
www.housewifeclass.com
@housewifeclass

Ordering Information:

U.S. trade bookstores and wholesalers, please contact HWC Press. Special discounts are available on quantity purchase by corporations, association, educators, and others.

About the typefaces:

Streetwear, designed by Artimasa (https://www.behance.net/artimasa)

Crafty Girls, by Crystal Kluge (http://www.tartworkshop.com/)

www.ingramcontent.com/pod-product-compliance
Lightning Source LLC
Chambersburg PA
CBHW060802270326
41926CB00002B/67